TRAUMATIC BRAIN INJURY

TRAUMATIC BRAIN INJURY

A Caregiver's Journey

Kim,
Thank you
for your ministry
of prayer!
Lydia Greear

Lydia Greear

To order additional copies of this book, contact:
Xlibris
1-888-795-4274
www.Xlibris.com
Orders@Xlibris.com
663969

Foreword

Caring for my family has taken me down some interesting roads through the years. I love my children. Having raised them on three continents, we are a close family. This journey with my son who has a traumatic brain injury has challenged and inspired me in ways I have never known.

Hello and thank you for reading this book. My guess is that someone in your world has a traumatic brain injury. After months of searching for resources from families who have gone through this journey, I decided to write. This book is the result of many months of walking through traumatic brain injury for my adult son, Thaddeus. Brain injuries can happen to anyone, anywhere, anytime. This is our story.

My name is Lydia Greear. My husband, Asa, and I have been married for forty years. We live in Palm Coast, Florida. We have three adult children, Thaddeus, Jeremiah, and Jessica. All except Thaddeus are married. Our family is bilingual. We learned French after working for fourteen years in the West African countries of Benin and Cote d'Ivoire and also in France. I began early retirement after twelve years of working for AT&T in May 2013. Six weeks later, Thaddeus was hit by a car and suffered a traumatic brain injury.

For Thaddeus, this is a difficult journey. So many things have been forgotten, and each day is a struggle to move forward. I managed his medical care and facilitation through brain injury back to independent living. For the last fourteen months, I have been near Thaddeus. He was thirty-seven years old at the time of his accident.

By his ex-wife, Thaddeus has two children—Holton Greear, daughter, twelve years old at the time of the accident, and Alton

Thaddeus Greear, eleven years old at the time of the accident. Thaddeus was single and, just prior to the accident, had broken off a relationship with his girlfriend of five years.

I am going to share with you a very personal journey as a family caregiver to someone with a traumatic brain injury. This journey was recorded day by day as we walked through the stages and phases of hospital ICU, hospital acute care, hospital progressive care, rehabilitation hospital, through Thaddeus's care at NeuroRestorative Community Rehabilitation Facility. These daily entries were first written on the dates indicated through the various stages of Thaddeus's journey to recovery. I am not a medical person. There are medical terms and references used by the doctors and nurses in reference to Thaddeus. We as a family learned most of them for the first time.

My research on brain injury uncovered the fact that brain injury occurs in the United States approximately every ninety seconds. Thaddeus was having a normal day, had met a new friend. He was heading home to play music when this tragic accident occurred. My husband, Thaddeus's son, and I were on a trip to Paris, France. Thaddeus had contacted us throughout the trip. He was happy and putting his life on a new track.

June 29, 2013

The accident took place at 11:30 p.m. in Lexington, Kentucky. Thaddeus was crossing in a public crosswalk at the intersection of Nicholasville Road and Malabu Drive after getting off a public bus. He was near the curb when a speeding small SUV struck him and flipped him over the vehicle onto his head into a perpendicular street. There was a young man with him that evening, and he saw the accident. He later described to us, "Thaddeus's body was laying in a pool of blood, and I was sure he had split his skull open." Thaddeus was rushed to University of Kentucky Medical Center, Lexington, within minutes of the accident.

June 30, 2013

In Paris, we were twelve days into a month-long trip. Our hotel was in a small suburb of Paris, Becon les Bruyeres, near the train station. We enjoyed a busy Sunday with friends at a fifty-year-anniversary celebration. All our cell phones were battery dead.

We got off the train and walked slowly out of the train station, recapping the day and talking about the next leg of our trip. We had plans to travel by car to the Touraine region of France. We were tired and headed across the street to our hotel. We climbed the antique spiraling staircase to our room on the third floor. We packed a few things to get ready for checkout the next morning.

Once the phones had a few bars of battery, we started received several text messages and voice messages from our daughter and son. Also we had a voice message from Alton's mother (Thaddeus's ex-wife, Allison). All of them were asking us to call. It was urgent.

We called Jeremiah, our son, and Jessica, our daughter. Each told us what was going on with Thaddeus. Jessica was at the hospital. It had been nearly twenty-four hours after the accident had happened. We were hearing the heavy news that Thaddeus was stable with life-threatening injuries.

As soon as we heard the news, we were stunned. In disbelief, we didn't know what to do. The only reports given to our daughter were "He is in critical condition."

The local police knocked on Thaddeus's ex-wife's door at 10:00 a.m. Sunday, asking if she knew Thaddeus Greear. His daughter, Holton, was at the door with her mother when the news was delivered. They called our daughter, Jessica, immediately. Five months pregnant with her third child, Jessica and her husband took their family to Lexington, Kentucky, and took charge.

In France, Alton buried his head in his pillow on the little corner bed, tears streaming and fear gripping his face as he thought he would never see his daddy again. I caressed his head and used my thumb to catch his tears and we prayed. Asa and I were in full shock! The words were playing over and over in our minds. We began to look for the news report on the Internet. We were asking ourselves what we should do. Still stunned, we sat for what seemed like hours.

The thoughts rolling through all our heads were about how serious this was! What had happened? How did this happen? Would we ever see him alive again? Would we be able to hold him in our arms again?

My thoughts trailed back to my last visit with Thaddeus one month before. Thaddeus had been at our house in Palm Coast, Florida, to spend time with me for Mother's Day. We had an amazing visit that week—walks on the beach, brunch at the resort, cooking and laughing together. He even helped me have courage to release my fifteen-year-old dog, Bibi, who was suffering from final stages of breast cancer, to be put down by the vet.

I remembered more details of our last visit. He and I had a very serious conversation in my kitchen in Florida. He told me that his life was changing. He said he was reading his Bible more. He said the words of the Old Testament were bearing on his heart. "Mom, I feel I am like the children of Israel. I have disobeyed God," he told me.

I had shared with him that he couldn't make changes in his life on his own. I pleaded that he needed to get help. He then startled me with a comment, "One day I'll just walk out in front of a car, and you won't even come to my funeral." I responded to him, "Well, first of all, I don't intend to go to your funeral because I will be gone first."

My thoughts were still running. *Did he do it? Did he walk out in front of a car deliberately?*

Asa and I finally picked up the phone and contacted the airline company and told them our story. A very sympathetic customer service agent took care of getting our flights moved to the first flight going from Paris to Cincinnati, Ohio. The airline was gracious, and due to the urgent circumstances, we were given immediate passage on the next direct flight to Cincinnati, Ohio, at 7:00 a.m. This was the closest they could get us to Thaddeus at the last minute. Our trip was over. We were headed back to the United States.

We packed up our belongings, contacted the front desk to prepare our bill. We laid our heads on the pillow for a few hours. With tears, prayers, searching, and hurt, we all three clung to one another, asking God to show us his way through this tragedy!

We contacted our friends in France to share the news. They began praying. One of my dear friends shared with me, "Lydia, tu vas faire un mauvais voyage!" You are getting ready for a very hard trip! She was right.

Our daughter, Jessica Stotler, posted the following on Facebook, Sunday, June 30, 2013:

Pray for Thaddeus Greear.

Got to hospital this afternoon. Spent several hours there. He is responding well. Just won't open his eyes. Thankful for friends who are letting us stay with them tonight.

Our son, Jeremiah, posted this status on June 30:

Pray for Thaddeus Greear.

Please pray for my brother, Thaddeus Greear. He was hit by a car last night and is in the icu. He is on a ventilator and responding to a point. Please pray for our family as mom and dad are still out of country.

July 1, 2013: Thaddeus in ICU

Asa, Alton, and I flew from Paris to Cincinnati today to be with Thaddeus. The hotel management was very sympathetic and wished us well, vowing to say a prayer for our son. There were still so many questions on my mind: "Did he do this deliberately?" "Who was with him when it happened?" "Is he going to change because of this?"

My heart was torn because we were just getting started on our vacation. Thaddeus needed us to be with him. We hurt so deeply. Denial, grief, and shock were all emotions at the same time. I was cool about getting packed, checked out of the hotel, and into the taxi to get to the airport.

We got checked in for the flight at Aéroport Charles de Gaulle. The agent told us we would be assigned seats at the gate. He told us they would take good care of us. A curious question he asked was if we had a pet. I told him that we did not have a pet traveling with us.

We went to have our last *petit déjeuner français* at the Paul bakery in terminal 2E at Charles de Gaulle Airport. Alton was excited to eat his two *pain au chocolat* pastries. I enjoyed my last double café, and we got through passport check without any problems. We were pleasantly distracted by a little boy in line who was teasing his mother by hiding and hanging behind. He had an Afro hairstyle larger than his body, it seemed. She was pretty strict with him, so he stayed close after her reprimand. It was entertaining to watch them interact. I remembered a little boy about that age who always tested the limits—Thaddeus.

When we got by Duty Free, I had to pick up a bottle of perfume. Our quick departure left shopping for any souvenirs to the Duty Free stores. It was a fun little stop, and then we headed to the gate. We waited a few minutes in line at the gate.

Then my altitude pressure started rising. I couldn't stand still. I was pacing the floor and fidgeting with my carry-on bags. My thoughts were racing from one to another. I wanted to run. I wanted to escape. I wanted to already be on the plane. I didn't want to get on the plane. Quickly I headed over to pick up a bottle of water for the plane, using up my Euro coins.

The gate agent announced our seats as he handed us the boarding pass—in the back of the plane! This triggered all kinds of emotions that had been so carefully held inside until this moment. I was furious. We were not really sure why the gate agent had done this. To me it seemed like she had a bad attitude. I was sure she was deliberately placing us in the back of the plane. She handed out about twenty stands by boarding cards. I knew she had messed with us. We spoke with another gate agent supervisor, who asked us again if we had a pet. Where was this coming from? We told them no. He told us that this explained our seats.

Boarding the plane was horrifying. The flight attendants promptly told us to leave carry-on bags in the front of the plane. They were sure there was no room in the overhead space. For me that was it. My cool exterior heated to boiling over at that point. I told her that we would not leave our bags. I ran toward our seats in anger. I threw my bags in the overhead bin and sat down. Finally it hit me—Thaddeus was in ICU and we were leaving France and I had seats in the back of the plane and I was mad!

I completely embarrassed Asa. In my seat, I sat completely still and shut out the world for a few minutes. Tears, fears, hurt, anger, and frustration were only a few of my emotions. Later after takeoff, I apologized to the flight attendant. She was very understanding. She told me that her job was to make sure I was comfortable on that flight, and she would do whatever I needed. I appreciated her gracious spirit. For the next eight hours, we got along great on the plane.

We arrived in Cincinnati around 2:15 p.m. As soon as we had cell service, I immediately called the ICU nurse taking care of Thaddeus.

She told me that Thaddeus was in critical condition. They had been able to stabilize him through the night after some procedures. Jessi began texting me, and we were trying to get off the plane. I just sat down and talked to her while other passengers deplaned. She caught me up on what was happening. She said Thaddeus was not responding to anything with gestures. She was told he had no broken bones. They had completed the CT scans but were completely focused on stabilizing him and treating the head trauma.

I breathed a sigh of relief because we had made it to the United States. Alton, hanging close by, hugged me, and I told him I was sorry we had to leave France. He said he was sorry too. He said, "Daddy needs us here." I agreed.

We got off the plane. I took a quick reentry photo of Alton and then headed to customs. It took a while to get through customs and pick up our bags. We picked up the rental car and headed to Lexington. We were in constant contact with Jessi and Holton on the trip.

When we arrived at University of Kentucky Chandler Medical Center, Jessica and her family met us! Thaddeus was in ICU on the seventh floor. He had been rushed by an ambulance to the ICU on Saturday night. The report she had about his condition said he arrived at 11:38 p.m. Allison (Thaddeus's ex-wife) was there with Thaddeus's daughter, Holton. Alton was happy to see his mommy.

We prepared to go into the ICU to see Thaddeus for the first time. One of the hospital chaplains met us. A St. Augustine friend had contacted Christine, the hospital chaplain at the UK Medical Center. She tried to prepare us for what we were going to see.

We stood outside Thaddeus's room. We took deep breaths to calm anxious thoughts. We were frozen. She went with us into the ICU room nearest to the nurses' station to see Thaddeus. Slowly and with great emotion, we walked toward his bed. He had so many machines hooked to him, keeping him alive. My heart was pounding, and my tears were stuck inside my head because of the utter shock of the sight.

He had blood caked in his hair, and his face was covered with dried blood, pieces of blacktop, and bandages. The bed was raised high, and he had multiple fluid bottles hanging above the bed. Monitors were framing his headboard, and the machines were breathing for him. We were told he was in a coma. It was standard practice with head trauma. The partially induced coma would assure he didn't wake up abruptly.

We held his hand, which seemed as though he squeezed, but we weren't sure he was aware. The nurses told us these were involuntary spasms. They said he was in pain. He was unaware of the massive pain because they had him on medications. We were only able to see him for a few minutes. Nurses came back in to chase us out of the room because they needed to move the lines that weren't connected correctly. We were told the doctors needed to add a heart line.

We asked for a doctor to speak with us. No doctors were available. Jessi went to find the nurse (Gina), who had been keeping her up-to-date on everything. She came to see us and explained what was going to take place. We were asked to step to the waiting room, and they would come get us when the procedure was completed.

We prayed over Thaddeus as a family. We circled him—Jessica, Asa, Alton, Holton, and me—each of us touching him. The medical team again insisted that we leave, so we moved to the waiting room.

Jessi caught us up on everything that had been done since she arrived Sunday afternoon. She handed me a stack of paperwork. She had taken care of everything up to our arrival. She had filled out admission papers and set up passwords for calls and kept everyone informed on what was going on. She was brave and persistent throughout the two days. I know she was relieved when we arrived and could take over. She was happy to hand me the folder with the hospital information in it.

My brothers, upon hearing the news, rushed to the hospital. They had tried to see Thaddeus on Sunday night. When they arrived at the hospital, the security team would not allow them into ICU. They wanted proof that they were relatives. Both of them protested, and finally, my brother, Hank, said they knew it was a lost cause. So they left. My sister Ro (an ICU nurse in Connecticut) had arranged for vouchers to use in the cafeteria. She was speaking directly with the nursing staff and giving us updates throughout the evening and promised to check on him in the night.

Jessi had her girls settled into the waiting room with their daddy. We found both girls in the corner filled with pens, markers, and pages to color among the backpacks of toys. She had things for them to do while she took care of running between Thaddeus and her family. Such courage and bravery on her part!

We visited with Jessi and waited impatiently until after 10:00 p.m. for them to let us know what was going on. I used the call button to speak with the nurses again, and I was told he was undergoing a procedure, and I wouldn't be able to go back. I protested to no avail.

We were so tired from traveling almost twenty-four hours, I had to leave the hospital and go to the hotel. The ICU staff assured me that they had our numbers and would call us as soon as possible. We checked into a residence hotel. With amazing generosity and support, this hotel gave us a better rate than my normal discounted rate. The list of hotels given to us by the hospital didn't offer the comfort and convenience for the price.

We had Jessi and her girls with us, and the hotel clerk, Debra, accommodated everyone for the night. As a family, we prayed and held one another. The journey with Thaddeus had begun, and there was no hope for the future except for the fact that he was still alive. Hour by hour, we sat and waited for news of the procedure until we all fell asleep.

July 2, 2013: Thaddeus in ICU

I woke up early (6:00 a.m.) today to head to the hospital and be with Thaddeus. We had no messages or calls in the night, so I was hopeful. We had carefully strategized to be at the hospital to speak with the night nurses before they left for the day. Asa dropped me off at the door before 7:00 a.m. so I could be there during the shift change.

I buzzed the door at the seventh-floor ICU 100's entrance. A young lady came out to say that Thaddeus was not there. Immediately I responded in panic. She said she couldn't tell me anything, so I asked her to please go back and find someone who could tell me something.

All my mind, soul, and body welled up at this news, and I was not very pleasant.

There is much confusion when a loved one is in the hospital ER. We are adjusting to the crisis, and everyday changes become major, dramatic events because of the unknown.

A few minutes later, a nurse came out and told me they moved Thaddeus to neurosurgical ICU on the sixth floor. I was confused and upset again! I asked why, and he said that the trauma unit on the seventh floor was to cover the entire body. Since Thaddeus needed attention specifically for the brain, he needed to be in neurology on the sixth floor. We clarified who the contact persons were for Thaddeus. We also assured that our phone numbers were on the list of whom to call. It is understandable that a busy ER could delay calls to family members.

I was upset and angry. I explained to the nursing staff that we trusted the care Thaddeus was getting and to please let us know when they are moving him. I left immediately and went to the neurology floor.

Arriving at the sixth floor, I was allowed in to see Thaddeus and his nurse. He had just come onto his shift and had no idea what was going on. I was upset. I got his name and waited impatiently for him to come back to explain things to me. We were finally allowed to go in to see Thaddeus. Understanding shift changes became a major point of education for us. The changes were from 6:00 a.m. to 7:00 a.m. Depending on how complicated the case, it could take longer.

Thaddeus was still covered in blood on his face and head. His was badly bruised on both arms and legs. He had a ventilator hooked up to him with a mouthpiece for breathing. His head was oozing blood from a brain drain that had been placed in the night before. He was able to squeeze my hand but not really consciously (involuntary movements are normal when the patient is comatose). He had movements on both sides of his body.

He had a line to monitor blood pressure, a drain tube to measure fluid overflow from the brain, bottles of medications hanging above him along with IV fluids, and a feeding tube going directly into his stomach via his mouth. He was unable to have a ventilator tube in his nose due to several fractures. We listened as the nurses explained what they knew about the broken bones in his body.

We sat with him all that day. Nervous and scared, I was fearful to leave him for a moment because they had moved him in the night without telling me. Asa checked his phone and saw a voice message delivered at 8:15 p.m. the night before from a Dr. Dillon. No one else had a call. We were confused because we sat in the waiting room until 10:00 p.m. waiting to see a doctor that night. No one had come to see us in the waiting room.

The ICU nurse found out what was going on, and I sat by Thaddeus's side the rest of the day until 9:00 p.m. They tried to wake him up every hour to see if he could respond by following simple commands like raising his thumb, showing two fingers, opening his eyes, or moving his toes. There were no responses to their commands. We were unaware of the normal protocols to check if patients are awake, like pinching the nerves in the upper chest. Thaddeus had several bruises from the pinching. The nurse was generous in telling us that he did not use that method.

Thaddeus seemed to respond at times by holding our hands. The reflexes of a comatose patient are sensitive to certain aspects of touch. Involuntary movements come from one part of the body responding to another touch. We just waited and prayed all day long. We were told these movements were not real movements—just spasms. We would be hopeful for a moment and then it was quickly explained away.

The nurses came in regularly to test his responses. They called out his name. Then they begin to tap his feet and arms. Then they pinched his upper chest. He was not responding to any of these things.

Someone from hospital finance came to see me about Thaddeus's medical bills. They wanted me to fill out paperwork on his insurance and potential payments from the insurance company for the car that hit him. I had no answers for them. They said they would send someone in who would help me file for Medicaid for Thaddeus.

A few hours later, a young lady came by with a large stack of paperwork to be signed and completed. She said she was with a third-party vendor sent by the hospital to assist us. She explained that her responsibility was to assist me in acquiring Medicaid for Thaddeus in Kentucky to cover his medical costs. I had no clue what this was all about but dutifully listened to her explain.

I realized that this had to be done on Thaddeus's behalf. He was completely unable to take care of these matters on his own. They asked if I had guardianship papers. I apologized and told them that I had only been in town a few days and didn't understand the term. She told me not to worry about that because since Thaddeus was comatose, I could make these decisions on his behalf pending the guardianship papers.

For the next hour, I worked through the entire stack of papers with the representative. I asked her if signing these papers made me liable for his medical bills. She assured me that it did not. She explained to me that we were both acting on his behalf, and once the ruling was made, Medicaid would pick up coverage for every one of his medical bills retroactive to June 29.

Confused and mentally exhausted, I really had no clue what I was getting into. All I understood was that Thaddeus needed help. I didn't even know his address before the accident. So many questions were rolling in my mind. How did this happen? What was he doing that evening? We remembered the last message we had from him about playing music at an event in town. He seemed happy that day, and we had been so pleased to hear about everything. Now we had to wait and pray.

July 3, 2013:
Thaddeus in Neurosurgical ICU

Early this morning, we went to the hospital to meet the night nurses before shift end. One of the neurosurgeons came in to report to us that Thaddeus had shown very little signs of change since yesterday. He said the drain would remain in place to monitor the fluids building up in his brain. Generally, these fluids slow down, and they would make attempts to clamp the drain.

That morning, an attempt had been made to clamp the drain, but the pressure built up, and that effort was abandoned. The team of doctors decided they would keep the drain until they felt he was stable enough to try again.

We were told Thaddeus was in a great deal of pain. When the sedation wore off, they would test his responses. His blood pressure and heart rate were rising. He was given another level of medication for minimizing detoxification. Also, they added morphine to control the pain. Those were working today. He could not open his eyes and did not respond to pinching in the upper chest or verbal requests.

These tests confirmed that he was still in the coma. We asked what drugs were in his system the night he arrived at the hospital. They said low levels of alcohol and marijuana.

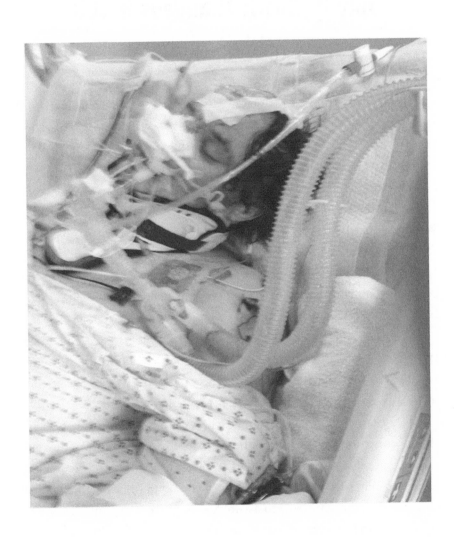

July 4, 2013: Thaddeus in ICU

Today Thaddeus had a fever. He had suffered tremors most of the morning. His neurosurgeon was concerned with the fever and the fact that his body was fighting furiously to ward it off. No seizure activity based on two EEGs. We were told that he had no further evidence of other broken bones but lots of soft-tissue damage.

Our excitement was overwhelming when the nurses made their rounds to check his responses. We were sure he gave us some indication yesterday that he could hear and respond to simple commands. I was with the nurse around 4:00 p.m. when she asked him to raise his finger, show her two fingers, and then squeeze or release her hand. He performed all commands with his right hand. Then it seemed he went back to sleep.

We were greatly encouraged, and the neurologist said that those types of responses were phase 2 responses, which she would normally see after the eyes were opened. He had yet to open his eyes. She assured us he was experiencing involuntary movement.

The brain injury can cause fever or a myriad of other possible things due to his injuries throughout the body. The brain drain would stay in place due to the fact that when they clamped it off, the pressure increased. He was breathing mostly on his own. They had him still connected to the ventilator to assure his lungs were opening up wide.

I loved the neurosurgeon quote today, "When all of his cells begin to connect together and he wakes up, we will see great progress." She had a positive outlook and had appreciated our commitment to pray for her and her team as well as for Thaddeus. We finally understood that the team consisted of the neurosurgeon's team of residents who were working in the unit.

Jessi and her family went back to Campbellsville this morning. She had been so strong throughout this ordeal. She stepped up when there was no one to take charge. Her enthusiasm and calm spirit had been amazing. All that she had done with two small girls plus being five months pregnant was phenomenal! That's my Jessi Starr!

Jeremiah had been staying close to us via Facebook and phone. It was hard for him to stay in Mississippi, but he had to work.

We are thankful for people who are praying for our family and keeping us close at heart! We were still waiting and praying by his side hour by hour. Many of Thaddeus's friends had called and stopped by the waiting room to check on him. We love hearing their stories of how Thaddeus was so loving and kind. Each had a story of how he had helped them.

This afternoon, we had a visit from the young man who was with Thaddeus at the time of the accident. He and Thaddeus had just gotten off a Lextran bus and were heading to the place where Thaddeus was staying. He described the people he saw in the accident. The driver was female and had three passengers in the car with her. She stopped and called 911 when he was hit.

Ryan said he had just met Thaddeus that day. Thaddeus was playing at a Lexington event, and Ryan liked his music. He said he was having a tough time and Thaddeus helped him. Thaddeus had listened to him share the story of some life problems. He had a similar family situation like that of Thaddeus, his ex-fiancée, and their two children.

After they had met, Thaddeus invited Ryan to play some, and they recorded music on his phone. They decided to go pick up another guitar and work on music together. Ryan said that Thaddeus was going to show him his method for guitar playing and record some music. Ryan was emotional when he told me, "I have played that evening over in my mind and wonder why I met him."

I shared with Ryan, "I know why you met him." Then I repeated what Thaddeus had said to me in the kitchen in Palm Coast about walking in front of a car and dying. I told Ryan, "God sent you to be with Thaddeus so you could tell us what happened. Did he walk out in front of a car?" Ryan responded, "No. It was raining and he ran ahead across the street. The car was going too fast."

We as a family owe a debt of gratitude to Ryan Hopkins. He helped us to understand what happened that day when Thaddeus was hit by the car. Ryan gave us words to calm our hearts. He remained in contact with me. There are no words to express what this young man had done for us!

July 5, 2013: Thaddeus in ICU

This morning, Thaddeus was not responding when I first arrived. He was draining more fluid from his brain today. His fever was lower than that of yesterday. We had a rough day yesterday with very little response and setbacks on breathing. The doctor set our expectations for this early yesterday. Her statement was "This is a marathon. There will be ups and downs, progress and regression."

This afternoon the tremors stopped, and they positioned his bed to have him sitting up. He is going longer and longer without sedation. The nurses were trying to get him to respond.

Facebook post:

> A few minutes ago Tatine, who works for housekeeping came to clean his room. She is from the Congo. We began speaking in French and she started telling me stories from the Bible about faith. As we talked we started sharing how important it is to praise God. We were sure he heard us speaking in French and he started raising his thumb and then two fingers.
>
> Before she finished cleaning the room we were both singing one of Thaddeus' favorite songs from our time at a church Cotonou, Benin, "Je Chante Comme David." We were dancing and singing together, clapping and praising God. Tatine was God's blessing to our room today.

One of my family members from Lexington brought me yarn and a crochet hook. I started crocheting squares I found on the Internet. Hours of sitting, I decided to be productive.

Thaddeus started running a fever. He was not responding. The nurses were trying ice packs to get his fever down. I stayed until the last shift arrived and then went to the hotel to rest.

July 6, 2013: Thaddeus in ICU

Thaddeus had a fever starting yesterday afternoon. The fever was controlled this morning. The suggestion was that he might have bacteria in the lungs. This is common for smokers and being on a ventilator for seven days. We were concerned about the fever. We were told that cultures would be taken and sent to the lab to see what bacteria they were fighting.

He had a new shaved hairstyle, which I was sure he would love. It is funny how my boys look more alike without hair. One of the ICU nurses was tired of seeing the blood and blacktop caked in his head. She started cleaning the wound and found another deep gash that had never been stitched up. Even after several days, it required stitches, so the doctor came in after we left and took care of it.

The doctor on call this weekend spoke with Asa. He explained that the fever was a natural process of the brain injury. That was the major plan of attack throughout the night.

Thaddeus responded visibly on his right side. These were positive. The left-side movements would develop with time. According to the doctor, he might be making some intelligent responses to us but would not remember these when he woke up. He was referring to Thaddeus responding to the West African French conversation and singing.

I was completely exhausted. Today I had to take some time away from the hospital to recover. Please pray for our continued strength. We had great friends who had offered a place to stay. The challenge was moving any farther away from the hospital before Thaddeus opened his eyes. We appreciate the UK Med Center staff and facility.

We rest in the fact that God is working all things together for our good. It is the power of God that will bring Thaddeus from the trials he is facing right now. We want to express many thanks to our precious sister and others who were posting great stories of faith in Thaddeus's life. I will repost these as I see them.

When Thaddeus was a little boy, he used to sing, "In my life, Lord, be glorified, be glorified . . ." Today the Lord was glorified. We walk forward in God's grace.

July 7, 2013: Thaddeus in ICU

We arrived this morning to a cleaned-up room and Thaddeus looking quite comfortable. He had a low-grade fever still that was being controlled by ibuprofen and Tylenol. There were some problems with his ventricular drain (brain drain), so this would be resolved or removed today. The pressure didn't seem to be building as much. We were waiting for results on the cultures taken over the weekend.

We still waited for him to open his eyes. He responded very little since Saturday. We were told the fever would set him back a little. He didn't seem to have nurses with a sense of urgency. We were not sure if that was a sign that he was getting better or not. We were so impatient and watching every moment for him to wake up. The days were getting long, so we prayed for endurance.

It was a long day today. Thaddeus had a friend come to visit. She had been calling and was quite concerned about him. The nurse had increased the propofol given to keep him sedated. This went on most of the day, and then she started weaning him down from 50 mcg to 40 mcg. We were starting to notice the medications he was on and the dosages—we watched everything!

Asa and I had to go back to the hotel to rest. Amazing how I just collapsed and woke up about four hours later. I was thankful to be at the Residence Inn. Asa was not excited about paying for a room. Personally, I didn't care. Comfort and security are important for me right now. Maybe in a few days I'd be able to change locations.

We had an eventful visit with the team of residents. They came by for rounds, and he didn't respond much. Then Asa called out to him and asked him to raise his thumb. He did a bold thumbs-up. Then he asked him to lift two fingers; he lifted four fingers. After that, he asked him to move his toes. We saw the big toe moving and an attempt to move more. After that, he was tired. Breathing was good, fever was down, and no bacteria showed up in the lung cultures. The doctors were not sure why he had a fever.

It was so hard to sit by and wait. I contacted my friends who had been prayer warriors with me over the last few months. They had no idea what was happening. I had to call in prayer reinforcements. Also I started sending out these updates daily on Facebook. Thaddeus's friends and our friends wanted to know what was happening.

July 8, 2013: Thaddeus in ICU

We have had a quiet morning so far. Thaddeus was still in a coma. There was still a drain in his brain to monitor fluid. At this point, the drain wasn't functioning and the pressure in his head seemed to be good. The doctors said they would remove the drain today.

He had been on a ventilator since he arrived. The doctors said he had to be transitioned to a tracheostomy. We didn't know when this would be done. According to the doctor, this would make it easier for him to breathe. Also this would avoid complications like infection in the sinuses, mouth sores, etc. I was googling tracheostomy and watching videos of procedures on my computer.

Thaddeus was actively moving his right arm. Yesterday we were excited when he responded to Asa's commands to give a thumbs-up and raise two fingers while the team of residents was here. He hadn't opened his eyes yet.

His risk of infection was still high because of the open drain and the laceration. Today he was not having any fever or indication of infection. His fever was almost normal after two days of antibiotics. They wanted to keep him calm and quiet to assure the healing could take place. This was still an hour-by-hour situation.

I remember the example of the marathon given to us by the doctor. The healing process will show waves of improvement and regression day by day. The true understanding of his healing process will come week over week. He didn't move his left arm as much as he did a few days ago. Today he was reaching for the tubes about his face with his right hand. They asked him to move his toes, give a thumbs-up, and open his eyes.

We continued to pray and wait. Alton came by to play his harmonica for Daddy. It is a hard thing for an eleven-year-old boy to understand. He had courage to come and see his daddy in the hospital. What a precious sight!

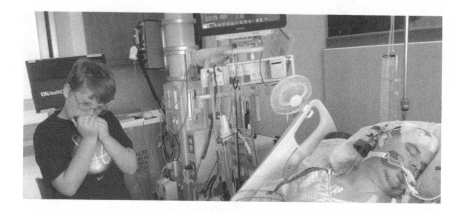

July 11, 2013: Thaddeus in ICU

This morning had been eventful already! We were excited to see Thaddeus try to open his eyes when we were talking with him. He had been responding to hand-gesture commands since yesterday. The nurse moved his bed to a seated position, and he was able to hold his head up and cough quite a bit.

He had a wonderful light-filled room. The blinds open and his bed facing the sun seemed to make all of us brighter! The nurse wanted to help facilitate his awakening from the coma! We were encouraged!

We were told he would have a tracheostomy and a PEG (percutaneous endoscopic gastrostomy) today. These would enable him to be weaned off easier from the feeding tube and ventilator. The procedures would be done in his ICU unit as we prayed all went well.

During our discussion with the neurosurgeon, she said she was encouraged by his movement and the consistent response to commands. She also explained to us that the tracheostomy would give him relief and allow for weaning off of the sedation.

Someone mentioned yesterday that he looked younger with his new shaved hairstyle. The laceration was healing well. We were going to work on manicure and pedicure next.

So many friends and family members are praying and walking through this journey with us. We believe in healing and know that great things are going to come from this experience. It is a long journey, and we trust God every day to bring everything together.

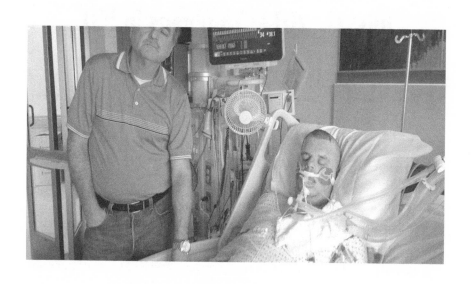

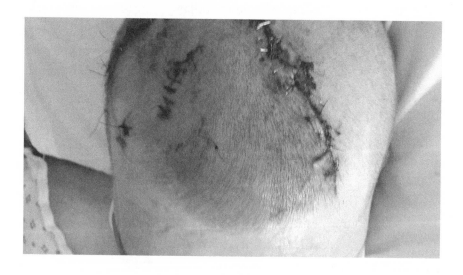

July 12, 2013 – Thaddeus in ICU

Good morning. Jessi was with me today. Thaddeus did well through the night. He had been consistently trying to open his eyes more since yesterday. The trach and PEG were not put in yet. We waited again today. Since he seemed to be awake, these would give him less restriction and less chance of infection.

Interesting fact: the ventilator has a tube placed in his vocal cords. The tracheostomy would be placed below his vocal cords, according to the doctor. He still wouldn't be able to talk to us for a while.

The progress for Thaddeus was steady, and we knew it was in direct relationship to prayers for him during these days. We are hopeful for his complete recovery. It would be a while before he was released from ICU. We had officially moved from hour to hour to day to day. Thank the Lord.

July 13, 2013: Thaddeus in ICU

There were interesting changes this morning. Asa and I bought Thaddeus a guitar and brought it to the hospital. We were told it was okay to place it in his hands. It surprised us that he held the guitar with his right hand as we held the neck of the guitar. Even with his eyes closed, Thaddeus was strumming the guitar to his own music and that of a French recording artist. We had partnered with the nurses to keep a watch on Thaddeus as they decreased his propofol this morning. I started playing Thaddeus's instrumental music on my iPhone, and he started strumming with his right hand.

His neurosurgeon came by during the jam session and was pleased to see what she called purposeful movement. Good news: we had progressed from involuntary movements to some purposeful movement.

We were seeing very slow and steady progress. We were told the tracheostomy and the PEG were still necessary. The ER surgeons had yet to put in the trach and PEG. We waited and prayed.

Asa and I were happy to have Jessi and the girls with us for a few days. Jessi was our rock right now. She would find out next week if she has a girl or boy. Stay tuned for the announcement. Juliette and her husband, Ryan, would celebrate birthdays on the nineteenth of July.

We want to say a special thanks to Crescent Beach Baptist Church for helping us with the hotel bill. God is providing for our needs in remarkable ways. We have a marathon ahead of us and are trying to keep the pace.

July 14, 2013: Thaddeus in ICU

We were with Thaddeus this morning. Overnight, he had the trach put in, and already he looked better. Also an MRI was done on his right knee. He had a new brace on his right leg this morning. Small phases of progress gave us hope. One of his nurses last night told us, "Any good changes will take time, the bad changes are fast." So far, his good changes were on schedule. God's schedule is our schedule.

Thaddeus seemed to be resting peacefully this morning. He had to have an oral feeding tube put back in for medicines. This was temporary until the PEG was done. Usually, both are done at the same time, but due to a busy ER, he had to wait.

We are thankful for people praying for Thaddeus and us. It was exhausting day by day. We were looking for a place to stay in for the long term. Since our arrival, we had been in a hotel. The manager had given us a good rate, and the staff had been accommodating. Asa was making plans to return to Florida next week. It was really hard for me to go far until Thaddeus woke up from all this.

Since our arrival, we had been trying to piece together what happened to Thaddeus. What was he doing? Where was he going? How was he emotionally that night? Asa was able to talk with the police about what happened on the night of June 29. He was told there was still no official police report because the incident was under investigation. There were some unanswered questions about what happened related to the driver who hit him. The information from the police and the young man who was with Thaddeus had given us a more complete story.

Recently, Thaddeus had been given some assistance from his church. One of the deacons visited with us. He said he had provided Thaddeus with a monthly bus pass. The deacon said he had seen Thaddeus three days before the accident. The church wanted to help him. He had asked Thaddeus if he needed food. Thaddeus told him yes. He requested that the deacon drive him to the store instead of just giving him a gift card. The visit was positive, according to the deacon. Thaddeus had told him about us being in France and spoke of what a great experience it was going to be for his son.

Another visitor who was with Thaddeus the day of the accident came by to see me. He said that Thaddeus had been playing music in the park in Lexington in the early part of Saturday evening. This young man was interested in Thaddeus's music and going through a really tough time. He had a break up from his fiancée and other personal hurts. He said Thaddeus helped him by talking through his experiences. When Thaddeus found that the young man was a musician, he had him play some songs on his guitar.

Thaddeus has been staying with a friend in Lexington for about six weeks. He contacted the friend to see if the two of them could come over and play music. That night they took the bus to the house of Thaddeus's friend.

The young man told us they played music in the bus terminal and Thaddeus recorded his music on his phone. Thaddeus made a phone call to a cab driver friend around 10:30 p.m. (I spoke with the cab driver.) Thaddeus sent an e-mail around 11:30 p.m. to his ex-girlfriend, according to another friend. The accident took place at 11:38 p.m.

At the bus stop on Nicholasville Road and Malabu Drive, there is no shelter, only a small sign indicating a bus stop. It was pouring down rain that night. Thaddeus and the young man had to cross Nicholasville Road over six lanes at the crosswalk. They stopped in the center of the first three lanes, and then Thaddeus ran ahead. (We as a family guessed that it was because he didn't want the guitar to get wet from the downpour.) He crossed the remaining three lanes and was almost to the curb when a small speeding SUV with four young adults hit him.

The impact of the car (young man said the driver didn't have time to put on the break, it happened so fast) threw Thaddeus from the curbside of Nicholasville Road to Malabu Drive. He was facedown on the street. He ran to help him. The driver of the car called 911. When the officer in charge of the area arrived, police were on the scene and had set up barriers.

Thaddeus was rushed to UK Medical Center. A passenger in the car was taken to another nearby hospital. The other three in the car were not hurt.

There are no personal effects for Thaddeus (phone, wallet, etc.). The police suggested that maybe these were covered in blood and put in a biohazard bag. These are generally incinerated because of the blood. The UK ER team didn't have anything for him.

We might have some more questions answered soon. How long before we had a police report? Did the driver have insurance? Were there distractions in the speeding vehicle (like drugs, alcohol, cell phone usage, etc.)? Who was really driving the car? (We have two accounts.) The most important thing is that Thaddeus is still with us.

July 15, 2014: Thaddeus in ICU

As I wrote this, Thaddeus was in surgery for the PEG (percutaneous endoscopic gastronomy) feeding tube. We had been waiting for this since Friday when they put in his tracheostomy. This would enable the nurses to provide his nourishment and give medications that were not injected. The delay was due to so many trauma cases coming into the ER over the last three days. We watched a YouTube video of the procedure, which helped us understand what was happening.

The doctors warned us that Thaddeus's recovery was a marathon, with good days and challenging days. He had been quiet since yesterday morning and running a fever. The nursing staff suspected that Thaddeus had a broken right leg. They had had a doctor look at the area and ordered an MRI. The results from the MRI came quickly and confirmed that he had a broken right femur.

The orthopedic surgeon told us he would have to have surgery on his knee possibly this week. There was a lateral and medial meniscus tear along with a break. We remained hopeful that he would heal and all things would come together soon. He still had a peaceful look on his face as he slept.

Jessi and Ryan went home last night for a few days. We were tired and keeping long hours at the hospital. It was hard not to be near Thaddeus when he was so fragile.

We are thankful for prayers and love poured out through comments, calls, e-mails, and visits. We listen to music and look to social media for contact with friends and family. There is a song that speaks of how

God does not delay in response to our needs. Even when chaos is all around us and we are unsure of what we should do, God hears and brings action to our prayers. The lyrics of Christian songs flow through my mind and bring peace.

July 16, 2013: Thaddeus in ICU

We were visiting with Thaddeus this morning. He woke up last night and had been communicating with his eyes, and we were getting pretty good at lip reading. He knew we were here, and we had been trying to tell him what was going on. The nurse had him sitting up in bed right now, facing the window. He washed his own face when she handed him a washcloth! It is the simplest of things that mean so much.

The neurosurgeon was extremely pleased with his progress. She said we were one day behind due to the PEG needing to be placed—all good!

Today he was scheduled for the knee surgery. The right knee was broken at the femur. The medial meniscus and lateral meniscus were torn, and there was a break in his femur. He had a piece of the broken bone attached to the ligament floating in his knee right now. This type of break is very painful. The cultures revealed an infection in his blood. He had been on antibiotics since yesterday at 4:00 p.m.

We were rejoicing to see him alert again! He had mouthed the words "I love you, Mom." Blessed my heart after so many days! That is our Thaddeus. Each day brought new beginnings for him.

July 16, 2013: Thaddeus in ICU

It was a new day in ICU this morning. Asa and I had officially hit the "weirder than normal" phase of this experience. We were exhausted, homesick, and reaching for morning coffee to keep these early morning starts to our day. There was a Starbucks near the hospital. Asa dropped me and made his morning run. Yeah, for Starbucks Rewards Gold.

Thaddeus has been off the ventilator and on oxygen since last night at nine. The doctor said he is still in post-op status since his surgery yesterday. They put a screw in his femur at the level of his medial collateral ligament. Here is the shocking part: the ligament was attached to the bone that was broken off. He did well in surgery.

Thaddeus is slowly becoming functional. I reminded the nurse that he normally is not a morning person. It was challenging for us to see such a previously vibrant personality slowly move forward to do simple things like washing his face. This would take some adjustment for me.

We were discussing his rehab in the next few weeks. Our prayer was to get him home to be near us in Florida. This is possible as God works out the details for us.

We were thankful that he was well enough for the surgery. We were thankful for the outstanding nursing care and excellent facility here at UK Medical Center. We were thankful that my sister is a trauma nurse and could keep us up-to-date on what we were dealing with. She calls every day and, on most days, twice to talk with the nurses. She supports me too! How blessed I am!

Evening notes: Today was hard. We celebrated the day Thaddeus opened his eyes. I must have expected too much because it frustrated me. We saw accounts of people in the media coming out of comas where they sit up, talk, and in some cases, leave the hospital. What a deception! When someone is recovering from a traumatic brain injury with other life-threatening issues, it takes a long time to recover. How could I deal with this loss! How could I deal with the pain of watching the slow changes? The nurses were telling me that patients don't even remember being in the ICU.

For me, today I focused on the things that I could control:

- My health
- My relationships around me
- Having a grateful heart
- Showing love and appreciation
- Finding time for my devotional
- Breathing exercises
- Exercise time and activity time
- Spending
- Positive thoughts

July 17, 2013: Thaddeus in ICU

Thaddeus was alert this morning. He had come a long way in a week. In order to help him connect again to the world he knew, we had been trying different things. We had been listening to his music. I placed my laptop on his lap to play his videos. He listened and, at one point, tapped the keypad. We tried a headset for a little while. It was too much, so he reached up with his right hand to take it off.

Thaddeus's neurosurgeon did a great job setting some expectations for us today. Her team was fighting the infection in his blood, and there were some breathing concerns. Before he moved to progressive care, he would need to have stable breathing levels and be able to fully follow commands without prompting, like "Raise a thumb," "Show us two fingers," or "Stick your tongue out." She said he would be slowly moving forward.

With this type of brain injury, patients revert to infantile behavior. This happens with most illnesses, but with brain trauma, it is more significant. This was what we were seeing with Thaddeus now. He was awake. He still had little to no movement on the left side of his body. There were waves of cognition. Sometimes he seemed to know we were here and then sometimes not. He was exploring his environment a little, reaching to scratch his head or pat his leg brace.

Each day he was getting better. One nurse told us to expect that in two days to two weeks to two years, he may return to quasi-normal behavior. He may or may not be as he was before. Only time will tell. In response to her words, we believed all this was in God's time, not ours.

July 18, 2013:
Thaddeus Was Mistakenly Moved Out

Thaddeus was settling down now after a very dramatic night and early morning. He was moved to a transitional unit at the hospital where they place patients who were transferred into the UK Medical Center from other hospitals. There was a need for extra beds in the ER and also neuro ICU. There was an urgent decision to take Thaddeus out of the unit to the transitional unit.

We were awakened this morning at four to the news that Thaddeus had been moved due to hospital needs for his bed. The move scared us! Unexpected and dramatic, this set Thaddeus back in his recovery.

We rushed to the hospital in frustration! Once we found him, the wonderful nurse on duty tried to help me calm down. It was tough! The room was dark, had no windows, and he was in a modified situation that seemed less than adequate. I was angry with the housekeeping of the room. I was demanding the doctor. Each hour I was asking where the doctor was and why we were not getting answers to our questions. The nurse brought me a packet and assured me that she used to work on the sixth floor neurosurgery ICU and had moved down to this unit because of her hours.

She said they had reached the doctor and she was on her way. After a few minutes, the doctor rushed into the room and demanded answers as to why her patient had been moved. She made a call to the unit and requested immediate return of her patient to the neurosurgical progressive care. She was much calmer than I was, but we could see her concern that he had been moved without notice.

He still was working through issues with his lungs and blood bacteria. He had been agitated with all the changes. His doctor was not able to get him to respond to commands. She had placed a priority with the nurse manager to get him where he needed to be for healing. We waited and prayed.

In the afternoon, Thaddeus was moved to a room in the progressive care unit. I was given the room number and carried some of our personal items up to the sixth floor. The nurses greeted me, and I was able to relax for the first time that day. No lunch or breakfast, we had been waiting for this move all day. Once Thaddeus was in the room, we left for the cafeteria while the nurses got him settled.

July 19, 2013:
Thaddeus Out of ICU!

It was a good morning already. Thaddeus was moved to the neurosurgery progressive care late yesterday. He was settled in for the night when we left, and we were thankful. His "homework" from the doctor this weekend was to be able to respond to commands by Monday. We prayed and waited.

Thaddeus had been on antibiotics for three days. His fever was at 102.5 today. The nurses had been trying to get this down this morning. They were taking more cultures to see what was causing the fever. We learned from the first set of cultures that these take two to three days. With the weekend, we might not know until Tuesday.

He was moving more on the left side of his body. We were told that physical therapy and occupational therapy would come by today. We had started talking with a social worker about where he would go for rehabilitation. Quick changes in treatment once they got to progressive care. Amazing how the simplest things began to make us feel like we were moving through this journey.

Today was the day we would have been returning from France. We would go again someday. My precious Muslim friend here in Lexington came to see me while Thaddeus was in ICU. She invited us to break the Ramadan fast (Iftar) at her home on Tuesday night. She also invited doctors to join us for dinner to answer any questions we may have. She prepared what I call Algerian soul food—olive soup, couscous with chicken, and a special Egyptian dessert with almonds and coconut. Thank you, my friend.

We appreciate the persistent prayers and the love shared with us over the last few weeks. God was showing us is mercy and grace. He was restoring Thaddeus little by little. The drama continued day by day. Mercy and grace were getting us through each step.

I kept trying different things to keep Thaddeus awake and see what he could do. Thaddeus typed this when I put my laptop in front of him on his bed:

\\\]\]/'../////"/""""
N,,,,,,poppkjojkkkkhbhnbnjjjkkmm,,nnnm
nmmm///koooolkmkkmmkkpoooooopoomkokk
p p p p p o m m m k P k k k o p o k p p p
[o o i o o i o p o p p o p o o k o i o o o o o k]
kkkkkoooiooolkkklkkklkoko0i[[

Family celebrations went forward during these days with Thaddeus. Today Juliette and Ryan had birthdays. Juliette is the daughter of our daughter, Jessica. She turned four today. We ordered a Teenage Mutant Ninja Turtle cake for her and Daddy to share. Her favorite Ninja Turtle is Donatello. I asked her why, and she said because he has a purple headband. We celebrated as a family. We had so much fun at the birthday party. We all wished Thaddeus could have been there.

July 20, 2013:
Thaddeus in Progressive Care

We were thankful for the support for us and for Thaddeus during these days. Facebook and other social media plus texts and phone calls mean the world to us. Visitors who had stopped by consistently to check on us made the day go better.

We were late in getting to the hospital this morning. I had an asthma issue. We were still very tired and knew there were many days ahead in this journey.

He was sound asleep at first. Once awake, we were able to talk with him, and he slowly responded.

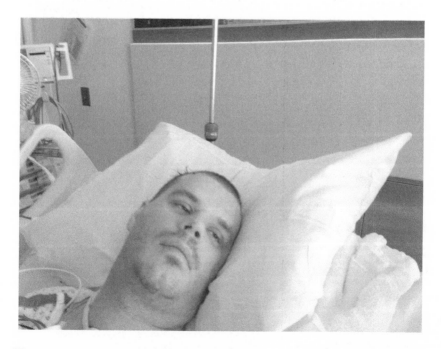

The progressive care unit is a step down from ICU. He had close nursing care (they had three patients per nurse), and the purpose was to help move him toward rehabilitation. He had been actively moving the right side of his body, and we were watching some reflexes in the left side. There was a problem going on with his left side, and he didn't seem to have control.

Every day we played his music to see how he responded. Most days he just closed his eyes and went to sleep. Yesterday he started moving his hand as if to strum a guitar. Then this morning, he mouthed the words to the songs. We had become very close to one of the housekeeping staff who was a native of Central African Republic. She came to clean his room and sang praises over him while she was working.

Music therapy came twice a week to see him. Yesterday when they came, they brought a tambourine and a drumstick along with the guitar they use to sing and play. The musician played some Neil Young songs that Thaddeus likes—one was "Old Man." Thaddeus reached for the guitar as the song was playing. We handed him the guitar we brought for him, and he started strumming along with the musician with his right hand. He wasn't able to hold the neck of the guitar but knew where to go to strum—small steps of progress.

July 21, 2013:
Thaddeus in Progressive Care

"Your love never fails. It never gives up. It never runs out on me." (These are lyrics from "One Thing Remains.") This reminds me that God's love is always present and he is working on our behalf. Thaddeus had to be restrained now because he was moving his legs off the bed. This activity was good and a normal part of his healing process. He was still running a fever, and he was at times delirious.

We were happy to have Jessi, Ryan, and the girls for an extra night with us.

Asa headed back to Florida this morning to bring our car back to Kentucky. He found out yesterday that his office was flooded from a pipe break issue. God was walking with us through every storm.

July 22, 2013:
Thaddeus in Progressive Care

We were happy that Thaddeus was responding to the doctor this morning. He was awake, and the nurses had placed a Passy-Muir in his trach to allow him to speak. The most audible words we could understand had been "My back is killing me." That prompted nurses to move him around in the bed some.

He had been restless and wanted to get out of bed a lot. These were great signs of the healing process. He had good reflexes and responded even with his left hand now. I asked him how old he was, and he told me after a few moments of thought, "Twenty-six." He still recognized Mom, and I had received a few appreciated kisses on the hand and the cheek.

This morning I rode the elevator with his orthopedic doctor. He said the surgery on his leg and knee was textbook excellent. He told me that Thaddeus would need to wear his brace for six weeks to assure healing. He was moving the leg from side to side and even crossing the legs. The movement patterns he had were normal with recovering brain injuries. While he could control the movements, he was very agitated and increased limb movements.

We were looking into rehabilitation centers now. Our goal was to get him to Florida for rehabilitation. Since we were not living in Kentucky, there were several concerns to work through. Thaddeus is a Kentucky resident. We are Florida residents. We prayed for God to provide the best solution for Thaddeus to go through rehabilitation.

At the present time, Thaddeus did not have insurance. There were higher chances of getting him into a program in Kentucky based on his pending Medicaid status. The nurse told me that patients who are involved in accidents and are from out of town have the same needs. We waited and prayed. We trust the Lord to guide us daily.

Asa's office was flooded. There were steps to take to repair the extensive damage. Asa had already planned his trip home. Then he heard there was a major leak in the office. I was on my own taking care of Thaddeus's needs. We relied on the support of our friends and family. Prayers were being lifted by so many. Some days on Facebook, I had more than one hundred followers keeping up with our journey. Deep breathing, crocheting, computer, and phone kept me busy as I waited by Thaddeus's bedside.

July 23, 2013:
Thaddeus in Progressive Care

We are thankful for prayers. Thaddeus had been trying to talk and moving his legs and right arm since yesterday. He attempted to get up and out of bed. He had to be constantly reminded to lie down and get well. This was our first experience with him trying to get out of bed. He seemed to respond to the nurses and me asking him to rest.

We thought he understood most things we said. He was trying to speak to us through the trach by using the Passey-Muir plug to create vibrations in his vocal cords. All these things are good signs of recovery. The final stitches were removed from the head laceration today. The scar looked good but still very raw.

The physical therapy team did come by to meet with us. They were supposed to begin placing him in a chair. Since he is unable to walk, they had to use a hydraulic lift system. There was a rubber-sheet-like mat placed under him. The cables were connected via large grommets on the edges of the mat. As they suspended him in the air, a therapist guided the contraption to the location where Thaddeus would sit. The mat was then lowered so that he was mostly seated and fully supported in the chair. He was placed in a chair for a few hours.

One of the goals for Thaddeus was to get him to be able to stand. The surgery knee was in a hard brace that did not allow knee flexion. His left leg was still not responding normally to commands. The therapists were able to place him in a supported stand next to the bed for a few seconds. The purpose of the session today was to assess his abilities and provide a safe environment for simple movements outside the bed.

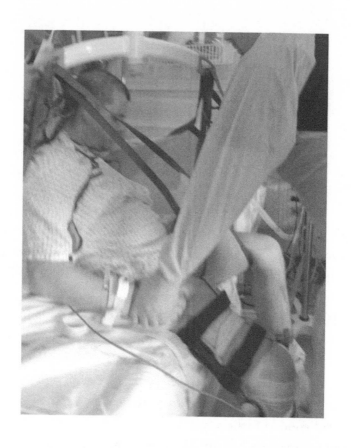

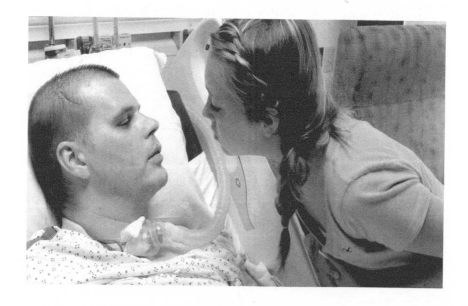

This afternoon Thaddeus was evaluated by a physiatrist (rehabilitation doctor) to determine if he was ready for rehabilitation. This was my first time to hear the term *physiatrist*. This type of doctor specializes in patients who have had trauma and require rehabilitation to return to normal life function.

Doctors were in agreement that he would be in rehab as soon as a bed was available. This was probably going to take place Thursday or Friday. There were lots of paperwork, evaluations, processes, and people involved in getting him ready for rehab.

We are thankful he is alert and active. The full evaluation of the long-term effects of his brain injury was weeks away. He had to be able to walk, dress himself, and perform normal daily activities. We were still on this journey for a few more months.

A group of musicians who played with Thaddeus prior to his accident told us they would like to do a benefit concert for him in Lexington in a few weeks. What a blessing to pay tribute to him. He has some really good friends who have prayed and stayed close at heart.

The University of Kentucky medical care is amazing. The hospital facility is state of the art. The doctors taking care of him are excellent. For these we are thankful!

During the visit with the physiatrist who works for Cardinal Hill Rehabilitation Hospital who came by for the approval rehab assessment, he introduced me to the Rancho Los Amigos Scale (a.k.a. Level of Cognitive Functioning Scale, http://www.tbims.org/combi/lcfs/lcfs.pdf).

He said Thaddeus was a Rancho 4 level brain response with injury to the frontal lobe. This is the definition according to the resource above:

Confused, Agitate Response. Patient exhibits bizarre, non-purposeful, incoherent or inappropriate behaviors, has no short-term recall, attention is short and non-selective.

He predicted the rehab would take at least one year. He would need constant care when he left the rehab center with many therapy sessions, doctor, and follow-up visits.

The following items were noted:

- He had a menton—reflex that moved his chin when you stimulated the palm.
- His repeated movement after the command.
- His agitation level and delayed responses.
- The responses that came and went were significant waves of movement.

He told me that lowered shades and soft music were important to keep him calm while he was awake. The rehabilitation center would provide a controlled environment with physical therapy designed to wear him out when it was done.

The meeting with this doctor left me with despair. The realities of just how long and hard we would all have to fight to get Thaddeus through rehabilitation were starting to set in. I had an appointment with a lawyer today. Actually, that was a good thing.

I left Thaddeus's room and walked the long covered walkway toward the parking garage to get into my car. I felt very alone. I couldn't stop the fear and the loneliness. I tried to call Asa. I sat for several minutes in the car. The desperation began to grow deeper and deeper. I became emotionally distraught yet could not cry.

I prayed in absolute desperation. "Lord, I can't do this! I don't know what to do or how to proceed in all of this. Thaddeus has no insurance, no help financially, and I just don't know how to handle all of this. I am being told I need to acquire guardianship to manage his affairs. What does that mean? How can I keep on doing this? He isn't Thaddeus anymore. How long will this take? The doctor told me to get a place to live in Kentucky. But I have a house and a life in Florida."

I turned on the ignition of the car and drove to meet the lawyer. I found his office through my GPS and parked the car. He was a kind and gentle man who sensed my frustration immediately. (It was probably not hard.) He took me to a conference room with his assistant and asked me some questions.

After a few minutes of discussion, he looked at me and said, "Here is what you should do." Then he paused and backed up a second. He restated it, saying, "Well, I don't mean to tell you what to do." To which I replied in all sincerity and humility, "Please tell me what to do. I don't know anything about what I am into."

With a reassuring smile and his pen to a legal pad, he outlined the steps we could take over the next few weeks. I was thankful! I asked him how much this would cost. He said, "We'll not worry about that now."

His assistant pulled up a copy of the preliminary police report. Then the bad news came for the first time. The small SUV that hit Thaddeus was not insured. Also, the police report declared that there was a male driver, not a female. All the passengers and driver were twenty to twenty-one. The driver had switched to the passenger seat. The car was impounded; air bags had deployed. Bottom line: we could not receive any financial reimbursement from the insurance company of the vehicle or the people involved in the accident to pay Thaddeus's hospital bills.

July 24, 2013:
Thaddeus in Progressive Care

Thaddeus was resting peacefully this morning. He had been taken for a vascular study to check for blood clots. He didn't sleep well last night, according to the nurses. I learned this morning that his care at the hospital would continue pending his approval for a bed at Cardinal Hill Rehabilitation Center. His needs assessment was in process. The vascular study was a requirement before he could be moved to a rehabilitation hospital.

Today I had more legal processes to take care of, so I was thankful for prayers as the lawyer and I worked together. Thanks to one of Thaddeus's dear friends who gave me great assistance in finding a lawyer. This man has prayed for and supported us throughout the entire journey. From the moment he heard about the accident, he had kept in touch with us!

This was day 25 of Thaddeus's TBI journey. We were weary from the journey and continued to walk close to God day by day. Yesterday I received shocking news that we would have to have a place to live in Kentucky for the next eighteen to twenty-four months. There were many challenges with this for me. We prayed for healing for Thaddeus physically, mentally, emotionally, spiritually, and relationally.

We were thankful for chaplains and pastoral staff who had supported us with prayers and visits during these days. We are thankful to friends and family who have provided laundry detergent, cakes for the nurses, snacks for the hospital room, hotel room payments, lunch out of the hospital, a dinner of fine Algerian cuisine, hospital coupons, connections with old friends, and even a car to drive. The people who had provided these are amazing and also deserve your prayers.

There would be a benefit concert for Thaddeus on August 2 at a local restaurant in Lexington, Kentucky. Through Facebook, Thaddeus's drummer from his band, Oldman Lowdown, volunteered her time and energy to provide this benefit concert for Thaddeus. Many thanks to Thaddeus's friends for their loving support!

July 25, 2013:
Thaddeus in Progressive Care

Today was a challenge day for us in making decisions for the future. Not being medical and being told we had to take care of Thaddeus after rehab was a challenge for us. We were praying for guidance.

Thaddeus was making progress slowly. He was alert but very confused. Physical therapy came in and had him on the side of the bed, lifting and lowering his legs in flex and extend movements. Normally, Thaddeus is very active, trying to pull himself up with his right arm. His left side had improved a little.

Yesterday he sat up in his bed and pulled out all his monitor attachments. It was a random movement, and we were told his body was responding to the brain injury with more involuntary movements.

We were told more about what would happen in the rehabilitation hospital. He would have a team of therapists, and they would have six thirty-minute physical therapy sessions per day. These would be designed to help him achieve more purposeful movement. We were not sure when he would get into the rehabilitation center at this time.

He was getting better at using his trach plug. Today they would do a swallow test to see if he could start to have water and ice chips. He was speaking French sometimes and English sometimes. He responded to commands and sometimes answered questions. He tried to speak often and spoke to his doctor in French.

At this phase of his functionality, he made some inappropriate comments. He frequently requested to go home, to get out of bed, to go to the bathroom, and today he told physical therapy he wanted to go back to sleep. He was aware of some things he was saying. When the doctor asked him a question, he couldn't remember he looked at me. He named his children without prompting today.

He was trying to find out where he was. Yesterday, when the speech therapist came for his session, he told her in French that he was in France. Then he turned to me and asked, "Pourquoi elle ne parle pas français?" I told him that not all French people speak French. He was okay with that. Then he told me he wanted to teach her French. Today he told the physical therapy guys he was in Africa. He started speaking French with Asa.

Asa made it back safely yesterday. We were trying to catch him up on what was going on around here. Some of Thaddeus's personality was coming through. He had to give Mom kisses throughout the day.

Every day was a new challenge. We were exhausted and somewhat uncertain on how to deal with this. We needed a plan for getting home. It was difficult to think of taking care of Thaddeus in Kentucky. God knows where we all needed to be, and he will guide us. We are thankful for our friends and family who continue to pray for us.

July 26, 2013:
Thaddeus in Progressive Care

Thaddeus was still speaking French and English. His nurses had a hard time understanding literally half what he had to say. We had conversations about going home, getting his things, and what time it was. Now here is how the conversation went:

> Thaddeus: I have to go home.
> Us: If you can rest and get well, you can go home.
> Thaddeus: I need to go home.
> Us: Yes, we want you to be able to go home so rest and
>   get well.
> Thaddeus: I want to go home.
> Us: Where is home?
> Thaddeus (after a few moments of silence): Je'n' sais pas.

At this phase of his functionality, he repeated phrases and stayed with the same thought for a long time. Then he moved on to something else. He could tell his nurses he was thirsty and needed to go to the bathroom. He was not able to get out of bed (it was a ploy to allow him to go home).

Yesterday, occupational therapy had him try to sit up on the side of the bed. He was able to sit for twenty minutes with assistance. Thaddeus was not aware that he couldn't walk and do normal things. He knew how to put on deodorant but didn't recognize a marker.

We prayed and talked with him. I showed him pictures. He looked at a picture of Alton, Asa, and me on the plane for France. He recognized Alton, and then I asked who Asa was by pointing at him. He said, "Daddy." I asked him again, and he said, "Mon père." I told him his father was standing next to him. He looked at Asa and looked at the photo. After a few minutes, he seemed to know that it was Asa. Until then he called him "Mon gars." Sometimes he thought he was a doctor.

I share these things to let you know we waited sometimes twelve to fourteen hours with him in a day. We always have one victory to share with you. It may come during a moment, so we embrace that one thing and thank the Lord. We found pictures and tried to help him make associations in our conversations. He could not stand yet. He was able to eat ice chips! Even swallow some water and watered-down Coke.

For these things, we were thankful. We went to look at apartments yesterday for my stay here. We walked one step at a time. God is good.

We are thankful for prayers. Our pastor in Florida called to talk with me. He reminded me yesterday that we based our expectations from what we saw on TV. On TV, when a person comes up from a coma, they are normal. In real life, when someone wakes up from a coma, there are months of recovery.

July 27, 2013:
Day 27—Thaddeus in Progressive Care

This morning Thaddeus was sitting up in his bed with the help of a large sling attached to a hydraulic lift. The lift carried him from lying down to suspension and then into a seated position. It was used to move him between bed and chair before he became too active. (Mostly he was trying to get out of bed on his own.) He could not stand on his leg yet. Plus there was a huge fall risk. He almost fell out of the chair even in restraints yesterday.

Thaddeus's neurosurgeon came in to speak with us. Earlier she saw Thaddeus alone, and he told her his name. He was also able to spell his last name for her. She asked how old he was, and he gave her the same age as he did for us—twenty-six. Two out of three correct responses are not bad. Yesterday he recognized Holton but still thought Asa was his doctor.

He was making progress every day. He had a setback yesterday because he spiked a fever. The explanations we received about the fevers were that there were many things going on with Thaddeus medically. The brain impacts the fever control center. He would not be able to go to the rehabilitation center until next week. Asa and I would visit the center today.

We were beginning to process some of the challenges we were facing. This was a life-changing event for us. In the beginning when Thaddeus's doctor told us this was life-changing, we interpreted that to be for Thaddeus. Now we see that this is life-changing for everyone involved in his life—parents, children, siblings, and friends.

Our plans for the next few months were unstable. It had become a reality that we would commute from Florida to manage Thaddeus's care until he was released from the rehabilitation center. The focus for Thaddeus was to get well.

We still had to set up a place to stay in Kentucky upon his release. He would eventually learn to maintain self-care. Until then, I would be helping him manage everything. The court date for receiving guardianship was set, and once that went through, I would have responsibility for managing his care and medical costs.

We were so thankful for the many prayers. We trust in God's perfect plan for redemption and love. He loves Thaddeus more than we do. To him be the glory now and forever.

Jessi (Thaddeus' sister) posted this comment on Facebook today:

> As I sit and eat a late breakfast with my little boy. I am thankful for all that God has done with Thaddeus Greear so far. He keeps protecting us as a family. I keep thinking of some prayers I kept praying to God starting in January 2013, concerning Thaddeus. I'm not sure why I starting praying it but God answered it literally. I meant for it to be figuratively. I asked God to drop him on his head, so he could change. While we pray for Thaddeus please pray for his total healing mind body and soul. Pray for a complete healing from addictions and a complete healing from his injuries. Pray that God will heal his soul completely. And remember when you pray for something to change or a person change, God might do it literally. Maybe this is the change Thaddeus needs. Just please pray with me.

July 28, 2013:
Day 28—Thaddeus in Progressive Care

Wow. It is hard to believe that we had been here at the UK Medical Center for almost a month. Thaddeus had improved greatly since the night he arrived. We had so much further to go on this journey.

After mostly talking out of his head, Thaddeus requested Christian music this morning. I was playing a song that talked about how when life is easy, we find it easy to praise God. Then when things are turned upside down, we sense God's presence with us, and when we get to the end of ourselves, we find God in a fresh and new way. As the song played, Thaddeus asked me to turn up the volume. Before the accident, Thaddeus was not interested in any kind of contemporary Christian music. He must have related to the words in this song.

He asked me if I could play the music like he heard in the Spanish church on Mother's Day. It is always interesting what he says. On Mother's Day this year, Thaddeus had said he wanted to go to church with me. I told him that I go to Iglesia Bautista Anastasia (Spanish service) on Sunday mornings. That day, Thaddeus first hesitated and then said okay. I had explained to him that the presence of God in the church is powerful. He asked if there was a translator, and I told him yes.

When we attended that service, the worship music inspired him. He was impressed with the worship team. He had turned to me then and said, "Mom, this is the real deal." I agreed! God always blesses through their music. I am so thankful that it lingered his mind today. Praise the Lord!

The respiratory team came in to clean his breathing tubes. They determined that he should be off oxygen because he was breathing for several days on his own without it. They said he had to keep the trach until after being transported to the rehabilitation center.

We are thankful for good medical care on his behalf. He was still moving and determined to get out of bed even though he wasn't physically able to walk. We had to keep calming him down. There were many inappropriate comments being made, and we tried not to worry about them. According to his nurse last night, this is a common thing.

Our challenges were many. Our hearts were broken. Our bodies were tired. The days were long. Friends were supportive. I was homesick. I love my son. God had given me a new mission in life for a while. I felt that I was in emotional "flexibility training" and not sure how well I was doing. I appreciated the prayers during these days!

July 29, 2013:
Day 29—Thaddeus in Progressive Care

We waited and prayed. Each day there was a new positive. Each day there were those things that made our lives challenged so much, we forgot the challenges from the day before. The cards, Facebook comments, and loving support helped us to maneuver to the next day.

This morning, we were looking through folders from the hospital given on day 1. There was a printed document on brain trauma injuries for family members, outlining what to expect and how to handle the stress of the situation. It is very helpful. Better late to find it than never.

Thaddeus had a great visit with his children, Holton and Alton. He called for them by name. Holton wrote messages on his dry erase paddle, and he answered her questions and read what she wrote. Alton brought his daddy a Mickey Mouse cap. Still very confused, Thaddeus responded to us appropriately at times. We tried to have conversations with him to make connections.

The benefit concert, Heart of Gold: A Show for Thaddeus, was scheduled for Saturday, August 2, at a local barbecue restaurant. The event was advertised on Facebook and through flyers and local businesses.

July 30, 2013:
Thaddeus "Graduates" to the
Rehabilitation Center

When I arrived early at the hospital, the nurses told me Thaddeus was going to the rehabilitation hospital. A bed became available. His nurse that day was a nurse we knew from years ago at our doctor's office. It was so good to see her again! She helped us get him ready to go.

Thaddeus had a traumatic transfer from the hospital to the brain trauma rehabilitation unit at the rehabilitation center. He was transported by ambulance to the location about five miles away. During the ride in the ambulance, he transformed from a neatly wrapped and covered patient to a wild and flailing patient. He had managed to pull down packages of sterile supplies with his right arm and put tubing in his mouth. He made it safe and sound.

At the center, the efforts to keep him unrestrained were futile. We were told that his confusion and disorientation would lessen as he progressed in recovery. The unit where he would be located was locked down for his safety. The admission process was simple with the prearranged paperwork ready for me to sign.

Thaddeus was taken by the EMT personnel to a holding area with nurses and doctors to monitor his vital signs. There were discussions about finding a special type of bed for him. We were given an overview of his rehabilitation program while he stayed at the rehabilitation hospital. His physical therapy, cognitive therapy, and speech therapy would all begin tomorrow.

Music therapy and Thaddeus's neurosurgeon were the top aspects of his hospital stay. Today was his last session of music therapy. The therapist had Thaddeus singing along with her on the song "Heart of Gold" by Neil Young. She played the tune and asked him to name it. He struggled, but when she started to sing the chorus, he sang with her. We invited her to the benefit concert on Friday, August 2.

His admitting physiatrist (a resident) came to set Thaddeus up with the bed and essentials needed for his stay. He explained as much as he could to make our transition smooth to this type of facility. We were given freedom to come and go as needed. We were encouraged to be a part of his therapy sessions. He explained that with his agitation, there would be need for restraints to keep him safe. Also, the hospital would assign a CNA—certified nursing assistant—to stay with him at all times.

He gave me some paperwork to read over about the facility and also some of the things we could expect while Thaddeus was treated there. There was a family waiting room near Thaddeus's room for us to go to get away for a few minutes. The nursing staff took his vitals again and introduced themselves to us. There were so many people involved in the process, we had no memory of the names.

Asa and I were exhausted at the end of the day. We stayed awhile with him at the center, but he was too confused and agitated to rest so we left him with the nurses. The doctor assured us that he would be at the hospital all evening. We were still staying at the hotel after more than a month. Friends had offered us a place to stay in a town about forty miles away. It was just too hard to think about being far away from Thaddeus. Their generosity blessed us so many times. We were unsure where we would stay for the long term.

We decided to go for dinner and then come back to see Thaddeus before bedtime. While we were out, the nurses released his restraints, and Thaddeus tore into his head wound with his free hand. They had called the doctor to look at it and then told us that he may have to wear a special cap to protect it.

Thaddeus's case manager came to meet with us. She asked about our housing, and we told her about our situation. She was so kind and helpful. We appreciated the professionalism and kindness shown to us during our first hours at the rehabilitation hospital. We had confidence that Thaddeus was in the right place.

Tomorrow would be a busy day for him. Asa would be in Campbellsville for a January Bible study training session.

July 31, 2013: Thaddeus at Cardinal Hill Rehabilitation Center

Thaddeus was starting to settle into his room at the rehabilitation center. The team of doctors, nurses, and therapists (OT, PT, and speech), along with the medical residents, would give us an idea of how long his inpatient care would be.

After not sleeping but for a few hours a day for over five days, he is sleeping now. The first rounds of assessments were done for him except for speech therapy. He just couldn't wake up for the therapist this afternoon.

I woke up this morning determined to look for all the positive milestones we had achieved. Finally, I felt the burden of all this beginning to lift. There was a long road ahead for recovery, and we wanted to get him to Florida as soon as possible. For now he was going to have to stay here, and so would I. It was good that I would be near Jessi and her girls, Holton and Alton. The Lord has built a wonderful support group around me as well.

We were still challenged with a place to stay for the long term. The options were there for us, and we prayed for God's mercy to find a place soon as Thaddeus healed. We were looking for a place with at least two bedrooms and handicap access. I knew there was the perfect place.

Asa would stay through early next week here in Lexington. I was going to go back to Florida for a few days. We had some friends coming from France for a short vacation. I planned to help them get settled, and then Veronique was going to come back with me to Kentucky. She is a dear friend we consider family. Thaddeus would be happy to see her, I knew. What a blessing. *C'est* cool!

Thank you for staying close to us during these days. I was blessed by a radio show this morning on WRFL Lexington. Sherri McGee (Thaddeus' band drummer) was guest on a live show to promote the Heart of Gold benefit concert for Thaddeus. Seeing Thaddeus's friends come together in this way is a treasure. We enjoyed a night at Willies Locally Known for several of Thaddeus's friends to come out and play tribute songs on Heart of Gold. Sherrie McGee had put together a large raffle with several important art pieces, guitars, jewelry, personal grooming items, and other music memorabilia. People bid on the lots, and with the entry fee, she raised money to cover medical supplies, clothes, and other personal items for Thaddeus. Each group, including the members of Thaddeus's band, Oldman Lowdown, had touching words of praise and recognition for how Thaddeus had helped each one of them. One of his artist friends sketched an album cover for a small compilation of Thaddeus's songs to sell.

Artists from around the Lexington area came to support Thaddeus. We were blessed!

August 1, 2013:
Day 34—Thaddeus in Rehabilitation

This morning, Thaddeus was alert and wanted to spend time with us. He was talkative with the doctors. He formally introduced us to the doctors. They asked him what time it was. He looked at his arm, and then we showed him a clock. He gave the correct time.

Each day was a new adventure with Thaddeus. He was able to sleep last night and wanted to get dressed this morning. We were hopeful in these positive changes. He got on a subject and couldn't seem to let go. He would ask repeatedly for the same things even if he got an answer. He had asked for water and food for two days.

I played the videos sent to me by his friends. He appreciated them so much!

We remained hopeful and looked for the blessings in each day. He seemed so happy to have both Asa and me with him today. He kept saying "Thank you." The doctors were looking for consistent patterns of cognition and physical improvement.

We still needed a place to be able to take Thaddeus after Cardinal Hill. We were looking at the possibilities to take him to Florida as soon as possible. Keep praying.

August 3–4, 2013: Days 35–36— Thaddeus in Rehabilitation

B efore I left for Florida on Saturday, Asa and I went to be with Thaddeus. We were there earlier than usual, and he was surprised. He greeted us and then said, "It's weird that you are here now." We spent time together, and I was able to let him know that I was going home to Florida for a few days. I told him, "You and Dad are going to hang out together this weekend." He liked that.

Asa was able to experience Thaddeus's first ride down the hallway in a wheelchair. The physical therapist brought a guitar with her for Thaddeus. He went with her to the gym to work on strengthening his left arm and leg.

On Friday we were given a place to stay. Gardenside Baptist Church had a two-bedroom townhome apartment for us to use. It was fully furnished with a washer and dryer. The social worker at the center put us in touch with them. They came to us and offered the apartment. We would provide a few extras—the basics we needed.

The benefit show for Thaddeus on Friday night (August 2, 2013) was amazing. Asa and I enjoyed getting away from the hospital for a few hours to meet friends and enjoy great music! Each group had a special tribute to Thaddeus. Tears of joy and relief from pain were sporadic throughout the night.

Sherri McGee and her crew did an excellent job. The wonderful words of encouragement blessed our hearts. We see why he spoke so highly of all his musician friends. New days ahead, and I took a lot of videos to show Thaddeus how much he is loved. I looked forward to the day when he would be back onstage and sharing his heartfelt thanks to them for this support.

I made it home to Palm Coast. Our precious friends picked me up from the airport. Other friends, who had been taking care of our house for us, came by to spend a few minutes with me.

My last activity of the day was to go to Anastasia Baptist Church to my church family. What a blessing! I was able to hear some of the great praise and worship music, great sermon from Walter West on conflict in the church from Acts 15, and then visit with my precious friends, Leslie Hunt, Janet Stout, and our ABC Single Professionals Lifegroup.

It was salve for my wounded soul and a treasure to know we have such a blessing in our church. Asa would stay with Thaddeus in Lexington. So many things we needed from God in these days. It is just easier to stop and thank him for what he is doing.

The center had to place Thaddeus on one-on-one care because of his agitation and confusion. Prayed he would be calm. Sometimes the nurses didn't understand his French, and it frustrated him. He had made it clear that he needed to get up to go the bathroom. This was a challenge since he had to be physically transferred by nurses and aides to the wheelchair.

Thaddeus was still confused and agitated. He said inappropriate things at times that hurt our hearts to hear. We had to be reminded that these things were temporary, and he was more embarrassed than we were that he had said them. Last night he told Asa he was sorry for what he said. It was so hard for him!

Thaddeus talked to me by phone and said, "Mom, my arm and leg don't work anymore." I told him, "You are getting stronger, and they will work again." He told me, "Mom, I am confusing my words." I assured him that he was getting better every day. Then he asked me to go across the street to his friend's store and buy him some cigarettes— you just couldn't help but smile. We said okay and then told him he didn't smoke anymore.

We are thankful for the dedication of friends and family to follow us and support us through this journey. We praise God, from whom all blessings flow in these days.

August 5–6, 2013: Days 37–38— Thaddeus in Rehabilitation

Thaddeus was making steady progress in his physical therapy. He was able to ride in a wheelchair from his room to the gym. The physical therapist was handing him a guitar to practice during each session. His left arm and leg were getting stronger every day. An x-ray of his arm proved that it was not broken. He had some deep-tissue injury that hurt when he tried to use it. Today he was able to stand on his own for a few minutes.

He was given mechanical soft food (shredded meats, pudding, applesauce, mashed potatoes, vegetables, and thick liquids) on Thursday. Now he was able to go to the dining room in his wheelchair to eat at a table. Thaddeus was eating everything offered to him.

Asa was staying with Thaddeus while I was away. He was able to get some of Thaddeus's belongings to take to the hospital. These helped him to remember his life and connect. It was challenging and rewarding at the same time. We rejoiced in small victories. Today we were told that he had at least five weeks of intensive rehabilitation ahead of him.

I was enjoying being at home. Our friends from France arrived late last night, and we had been enjoying the sunshine. Each day had a new opportunity.

August 7–9. 2013: Days 39–41— Thaddeus in Rehabilitation

Thaddeus was making steady progress daily. Asa came home to Florida last night, and I was on my way to Lexington. We would be living like this for several weeks.

He had good days and bad days. He had no regular pain but many inconveniences related to his left side being so weak. Daily, his physical therapy and speech therapy proved beneficial. There were activities for him to complete in his room. He was able to stand again and seemed quite pleased to be able to accomplish such a monumental task.

Today I spoke with his nurse by phone. She removed the stitches from his leg, and the wound was healing well. His aid was able to take him for a stroll in the wheelchair to sit in the sun. Wow! We are thankful for small blessings that mean so much.

Thaddeus had been quite agitated and wanted to now remove his feeding PEG. When he became confused and agitated, it made him miserable. Some days, he still didn't know Asa. Yesterday he talked to me by Asa's phone and asked me to give Asa a message. I told him okay. He asked when I was coming back. I told him that I would be back today. He told me to hurry up.

All our grandchildren started school this week. Ary was enjoying her teachers and had made some friends. Holton and Alton are busy in middle school. Juliette was enjoying her time with Mommy but missed Ary for not being there.

Chelsi was hired to work at the early childhood program she applied for a few months ago. This had been a constant prayer request for months. Good news in the middle of our struggles!

I had enjoyed my time at home. It helped to sleep in my own bed and find familiar surroundings. When I arrived at home last week, it was a weird experience. My heart and mind had been so engaged in Thaddeus and his care that I thought I lost myself somewhere.

Our friends from France arrived Monday night after a long travel experience from Paris. It was great to have them here right now. We have been lifelong friends since our first trip to France in 1987. Our visits with them yearly have been a blessing. This year, they decided to come to spend their vacation in Florida. Pascale and Veronique were just young ladies working in the day care in those days. Pascale has two daughters, Clemence and Mathilde. It was great to see them!

I was able to show them around Palm Coast and St. Augustine. Yesterday we went to Disney for the day. I am impressed that we could do three parks in one day—Magic Kingdom, Epcot, and Hollywood Studios.

Disney always makes me smile, and riding the Thunder Mountain Railroad with a special young lady, Clemence, made me smile even more! What fun! The girls taught me about the Pirates of the Caribbean boat ride, and it was also fun!

Veronique and I traveled back to Kentucky together. She has been keeping in touch with us via e-mail and

August 10. 2013:
Conversation with Thaddeus

Thaddeus: Hello, I need you to get me out of here.

Me: Okay, who am I?

Thaddeus: You are my friend.

Me: What is my name?

Thaddeus: Uh . . . uh . . . uh, I am not sure.

Me: Mom.

Thaddeus: I need to call Mom so she can pick me up tomorrow.

Me: I am Mom.

Thaddeus: No, I need Mom.

Me: I am Mom.

Thaddeus: I know. I need to talk to Mom.

Me: Who am I?

Thaddeus: You are Molly.

Me: No, I am Mom.

Thaddeus: Mom, I need you to pick me up tomorrow.

Me: What time?

Thaddeus: Uh . . . uh . . . uh, two o'clock.

August 10–11, 2013: Days 42–43— Thaddeus in Rehabilitation

Thaddeus knew Veronique as soon as he saw her. He had an interesting conversation with her about some of his favorite French authors, Flaubert and Camus. I was surprised by all this! He started talking about a book that he read with Jeremiah, *The Gambler* by Fyodor Dostoyevsky. His mind is an interesting place. He traveled a lot in his mind these days. He was in France while Veronique was talking to him. Then today he went to Texas after he went to Kansas. At some point in his life, he had spent time in these places.

Today we took him outside twice. It was he first time he went to the front porch for about one minute and he asked us to take him back to the room. He ate lunch and dinner in the assisted dining room. He was able to put a little bit of weight on his left leg. It was very weak.

We enjoy his humor. He will say something jokingly and have all of us laughing as he cracks a smile. Prayers keep us going. He prays too. He prayed for peace and safety. He asked God to get him out of the hospital. When we prayed with him, he became quiet and then rested.

August 14–15, 2013: Days 44–45— Thaddeus in Rehabilitation

It was hard to sit by and watch day after day when Thaddeus was not sure where he was and what was going on. He was in Macon, Georgia, when he woke up yesterday. His girlfriend was Julie. He was looking for Robert, the man he worked for on rooftops in those days.

Every day I reminded him what day it was, where he was, and what happened. He didn't know me at first yesterday. After a few hours of discussion, he finally gave in, "I'll call you Mom then." We went for a wheelchair ride to the garden to sit in the sun. He relaxed and seemed to enjoy being outside.

His pastor, Todd Lester, came for a visit. He had active conversation with him about how he was praying to God every day. He told Todd a story about how a man was preaching to him at church. He went to the man and told him that it was amazing how he spoke directly to him. The man responded by saying that it was the Holy Spirit speaking to him in the message. Then he realized that Todd was the preacher.

From that point on, he knew I was Mom and stepped into reality for a little while. His speech therapy, physical therapy, and occupational therapy sessions kept him busy all afternoon. We had lunch and dinner together (his mechanical soft food and me encouraging him to eat).

Every afternoon, he became confused and fearful. The fatigue level played into this. He kept trying to go home. This kept the nurses and aides answering call buttons. His routines were becoming steady. We were watching for him to become consistently coherent in his conversations and movement. This would take time.

Today the team of doctors and physical therapists would meet to discuss his progress and his plan for the next few weeks. We depended on their expertise to show us the right way.

Yesterday, I met some of the church members who were cleaning the apartment next to mine. They were so loving, they offered to complete anything that was missing or needed. I asked where I could find a gym. One lady showed me how to get to the YMCA. They needed an instructor, hmm. I decided that workouts would help me cope and find a sense of normal life. Thanks, Diane.

My prayer for Thaddeus: "O you afflicted one tossed with tempest, and not comforted, behold, I will lay your stones with colorful gems, and lay your foundations with sapphires" (Isa. 54:11). "He will bring me forth to the light; I will see His righteousness" (Mic. 7:9).

August 16, 2013: Day 45— Thaddeus in Rehabilitation

Today it was a little cooler outside here in Lexington, Kentucky. Thaddeus and I went for a walk in the garden after his physical therapy and occupational therapy sessions. We talked to Asa and Jessi by phone. Thaddeus was using his left hand more and more. It seemed he had better range of motion in his shoulder as well.

The doctor was changing his medications to help his brain heal faster. We were warned that he might have more agitation and disorientation. I told her I would stand by to assist as much as possible.

When we got back from our wheelchair stroll, he wanted to rest. They got him back into bed, and he told me this, "Hearing the words from your mouth are important to me. Just hearing you and Dad talking is important. I was talking to Bart the other day, and I told him that I was listening to you and Dad talking, and it meant the world to me. He asked me what you said, and I told him it didn't matter— just hearing you talk to one another set my heart on fire." (Bart is my brother. He had not been able to speak to Bart since the accident.)

Day by day he was stronger. We prayed his brain would heal and he would always know where he was. When I met Thaddeus coming from physical therapy today, he said that he was in a hospital. I told him it is a good hospital.

I was looking for positives in every day. "The joy of the Lord is my strength"

(Neh. 8:10).

August 15, 2013: Day 46—
Thaddeus in Rehabilitation

Thaddeus has had two days of important physical therapy. This morning, he walked between the parallel bars for the first time since the accident. He was able to do this with much assistance from the physical therapists. With the broken right leg (his strong leg), the task would take time to accomplish on his own.

We went to the conservatory, where I played the piano for him. He enjoyed the music and was able to focus for about half a song. Then we sat down to rest a few minutes. The time was slowly passing, and his accomplishments were minimal. We were thankful for progress.

Thaddeus spent much time in prayer. He would close his eyes for a few minutes, and I asked if he was okay. He said, "Yes, I am praying." It helped him. He was asking God to help him not to drink anymore. He was asking God to protect him every day and give him peace.

The garden here had green beans, tomatoes, squash, corn, and eggplant produce right now. He was a little interested when we walked through. He was more interested in the lavender, basil, thyme, and mint. His sense of smell is strong.

We made two trips to the garden today, picking a green bean, a tomato, and a handful of fresh herbs.

The next step was Thaddeus and his physical therapists would be going out for breakfast at a restaurant. If he was cleared to go, I would accompany them on his outing.

August 16–17, 2013: Days 47–49 — Thaddeus in Rehabilitation

There had been some eventful days this week for Thaddeus. I am sure we had passed from the day to day to the week by week. Thaddeus's physiatrist told me we were in for many months of recovery. I kept hearing that, and now it was starting to sink in.

The few steps he made on the left leg have somehow caused him to want to use that leg more often. Great news for helping him get out of bed and to the bathroom. He also used his left arm more.

The physical therapy team took four patients to breakfast on Friday morning (yesterday), and Thaddeus was one of them. Each patient was loaded into the transport vehicles with their wheelchairs. One PT per patient drove across town to the First Watch Café in Lexington. I followed behind in my car to enjoy the event!

Thaddeus was on his first outing since the accident.

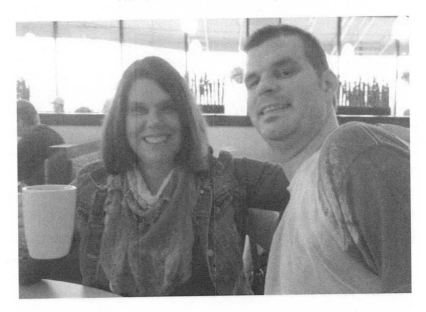

Thaddeus did so well. He was pleased to be out but was a little tired at some points. He was able to order his chocolate chip pancakes from the menu. We selected a side of scrambled eggs for him. He was able to hold the fork in his left hand while he cut his pancakes with the right hand using a knife. This lasted through a third of his large pancake. The scrambled eggs were easier to eat.

I took pictures.☺ It was awesome to be out with him. He wanted me to put him in my car and go home. So it took some convincing to help him understand that he had to go back to the hospital. Fantastic physical therapy program!

Thaddeus was relearning everything these days. He has always been a talker, so talking is no problem for him. Whatever came into his mind, he said in French or English. It was as though his entire life had been broken apart into small pieces like those of a huge jigsaw puzzle. Every day, new pieces of his life came through. The large jumbled jigsaw puzzle will one day become a clear picture for him. There are a few confused connections.

He spoke of people as though an event just took place or was going to take place. It was a sad moment when Thaddeus asked me, "Where is Momaw?" I told him that she is in heaven with Jesus, singing. He looked at me confused, and I told him she had died. He hung his head for a few minutes.

It was hard for Thaddeus. He wanted to leave, then when he was out, he wanted to go back to bed. His attention span was longer. Maybe he could focus for about three to five minutes. In the morning, after a good night's sleep, he spoke clearly and seemed to understand most things. Then throughout the day, he became tired and, finally, agitated and confused.

I left him in the doctor and nursing care with his aunt Pat on guard this weekend. It was hard to step away. Our friends from France, Veronique, Pascale, and her girls, left for Paris at noon. One more day to rest, and then I went back for another stretch.

August 20, 2013:
Day 50—Thaddeus in Rehabilitation

Live from sunny Palm Coast, I was resting and writing an update for you. These days were precious for me to be able to recover a little from the emotional and physical stress of walking through the journey with Thaddeus.

Asa's sister, Pat Estep, was on Thaddeus's bedside, encouraging through the day while I was here. Holton and Alton were able to visit him today. He remembered some people at certain times, but not everyone. The confusion was hard to understand for all of us.

Sometimes Thaddeus would crack a joke. We saw his sly smile and laughed. He wanted so much to get well and get out of the hospital. That was what it took to move him forward. He was clean and sober and without cigarettes for fifty days now. God is good.

As God speaks to his heart and mind, we believe we will see a new day and a future for him. "Call to me and I will answer you, and will tell you great and hidden things that you have not known" (Jer. 33:3). He told me that we were being attacked and that God would help us through the battle. Amen, Thaddeus.

August 21–23, 2013: Days 51–53—
Thaddeus in Rehabilitation

I made it back to Lexington on Monday to find that Thaddeus had fallen while getting into his wheelchair on Sunday. He did not hit his head during the fall. He was too quick for the nurse who did not lock his wheelchair when he was getting into it. It was a continual challenge to assure he has good nursing care. This made it hard for me to step away.

Thaddeus was happy to see me. His physical therapists took him to the conservatory to play the piano. He used his right hand easily but still struggled to use the left hand when playing his blues.☺ He had a busy day and seemed to be doing quite well in his improvements physically.

On Tuesday, the medical team met to determine his progress and how much longer he was projected to be in rehabilitation. We were still on track for three more weeks here. Based on their assessments and discussion, he was moved to a new room closer to the nurses' station. This would allow him to have more freedom and a nurse to stay close to him. His knee was swollen, and he had to have another X-ray. The bone was growing in a deformed fashion, and that pushed into the soft tissue. They told me this is normal for brain trauma and broken-bone healing.

The music therapy team from UK Hospital was able to get permission to come to Thaddeus yesterday. He was happy to see them and also sing along while they played music. This was the first time Chris and Jessi were able to come into this hospital to work with a patient. We were excited to help open this new door.

I had to meet with security again because of the robbery in Thaddeus's first room here. For some reason they had discounted my report of having money stolen. It was tough enough to deal with the violation of someone getting into my purse while we were five doors away in the patient dining room. I was very upset to find they thought I was "exaggerating" the event. I felt my integrity was questioned. The head of security met with me. He had been given wrong information by the staff. My police report was documented.

You can see that this journey became stranger every day. Good things were happening, and it seemed there were attacks that continued to challenge us. Please continue to pray for us.

August 24, 2013: Day 54— Thaddeus in Rehabilitation

Great start to the day with Thaddeus. He was alert and talking about things that happened yesterday when I arrived this morning. During physical therapy and occupational therapy, he wanted me to play some Ted Nugent. ☺ Then they put him up to use the walker for a few steps. He went around the PT gym with the assistance of three PTs. Music always motivates him.

The reality of having four more weeks, another knee surgery, and months of rehabilitation kind of had me in a funk today. Thank goodness Asa was going to be here Sunday evening. There were miles to go, and each new step meant we were heading in the right direction. I prayed I could find some fun in each day.

The apartment was working out well for now. Thanks to Shirleen Maynard, who brought me some needed household items (storage bowls, linens, and a room freshener). I am thankful for Allison and Holton coming to spend the evening with us yesterday. He told me I could publish some photos. I am thankful for prayers and those of you who continue to let me know you are praying. God is faithful.

I prayed we could get Thaddeus to Florida as soon as possible. We believed God would work this out for us.

August 25, 2013: Day 55—
Thaddeus in Rehabilitation

Thaddeus had been in rehabilitation for three weeks. His progress was excellent with steady improvements. He had less agitation throughout the day. The evenings were hard because he became confused. He didn't know who I was or where he was.

Asa and I were trying to put things in place for the long term. Being here alone with him was the hardest thing to endure. When crisis first hits, many people are near. Then the days become long, and the support lessens. We were still in the midst of the battle.

Our focus of prayer for healing was his brain and also his right leg. The bone was growing toward the sciatic nerve in the back of the leg. The casing of the bone would place pressure, potentially causing numbness and pain. For now, the physical therapists would focus on his ability to keep the leg stretched.

Wednesday night, a nurse's aid (no badge) came when we placed a call to the nurse to take him to the bathroom. She was rude and treated Thaddeus with disrespect. She huffed and puffed as she got someone to help her take him to the bathroom. She was yelling at him because he didn't do what she told him to do. She kept being disrespectful, and at one point, he looked at me and wanted help. He was upset that we had called the nurses to help him. He could not urinate.

She came back with a sign in large red lettering stating "Next bathroom time is 9:30 p.m." She said he really didn't know when he needed to go. He told me that he had a hard time going with her. He was put into bed. I left the hospital at 9:00 p.m.

When I returned at 7:40 a.m., the sign was still on the paper towel dispenser, stating that his next bathroom time was 9:30 p.m.

At dinner on Thursday, Thaddeus was not given any liquids except milk. We asked for water. He was not able to tolerate regular water, so he got the Nectar lemon drink or thickened juices. When we asked for drinks, he was brought thickened iced tea and milk. Tara worked with Thaddeus until 11:00 p.m. We asked for something to drink. We were told that there was only iced tea. No one offered to provide a thickened noncaffeinated beverage. He was given four cups of premixed thickened iced tea for the evening. I left at 10:15 p.m. after he was showered and had a new gown to sleep in.

When I came back this morning at seven thirty, he had been completely changed in the night. I was told he had an incontinence issue.

Today his speech therapist was sick and cancelled at the last minute. Then the nursing staff was short, so they couldn't take him to the toilet or help him. I became so frustrated and upset that he had no nursing care that I had to step away. It became too much to watch, and I was helpless in getting him around from bed to toilet, etc.

Friends Carlos and Joni Cracraft came and took me to lunch. It was a treat to be out with normal people. I appreciated the fellowship more than the steak. Each day was challenging. My heart was weary. I was lonely. I was sad. I was challenged on every side. I prayed to find help and peace. Only God could relieve my suffering and make this look right.

August 25–26, 2013: Thaddeus in Rehabilitation

The days were long for Thaddeus and me. He was able to make a few steps in physical therapy on the walker on Thursday. The cool thing was that it made him aware of his legs and how to use them. Now he wanted to be more mobile and had to be restrained and watched after. He was using his left arm better. He could lift milk during his meal to drink.

His brain challenges were related to being able to put memories together. He remembered many different things that had happened throughout his life. Sometimes he would tell about an event that combined different places, people, and situations. I tried to help him put the pieces together.

We played simple card games, and he could last about six minutes now before he got tired. For the last two days, we had no music, no television, and I had even tried some movies, but he couldn't watch them.

Challenges with nursing care seemed to be aggravated each day. I met with hospital administration after his second fall in a week. I kept praying for these things to be resolved.

Asa would be arriving tomorrow evening to stay with us. Thaddeus had been looking for Asa, Jessi, and Jeremiah. He responded so positively every time I came into the room. Carlos and Joni Cracraft came by yesterday to take me to lunch, and he was completely alert during their visit. After we came back, he couldn't remember their visit and didn't know who I was again. This was a regular daily occurrence for a few minutes. Then it went back.

Today he had a visit from James and Pat Estep (Asa's sister). He was happy to see them and knew who Pat was for most of the visit.

We are thankful for prayers. We look for blessings in each day. Today we were thankful for Pat's visit. ☺

August 27, 2013:
Day 57—Thaddeus in Rehabilitation

Asa and I had been visiting with Thaddeus together today. The last few days, he had struggled with sadness in the mornings. After a few minutes of conversation, he wakes up and gets some energy. When he saw Asa last night, he raised his hands in praise to God for bringing him here. We appreciated the return of his personality even if just for a few minutes. Hopefully, these minutes would get longer and more consistent.

We received news today that Thaddeus's PEG (feeding tube) would be removed on Wednesday. Due to the potential for bleeding, the doctors left it in for six weeks.

We told him this news, and he said, "The one Pawpaw put in me? Jeremiah pulled it out the other day and showed it to me. I just put it back." Yeah, sometimes he was confused.

Thaddeus had been on medication to stimulate his brain for a week. The new medications would now increase his memory function. He responded well to the drug therapies used to help heal the brain. We are thankful for all the prayers!

Asa Greear's Facebook post:

> Arrived in Lexington last night found Thaddeus to be sweet responsive and praising God for my arrival "Dad when are you going to get me out of here." His short term memory is still not connecting. He is responding

well to all treatments you all are praying and God is working. Lydia is getting much needed rest this morning. Thaddeus and I read psalm 20 together and prayed this morning God is working.

August 28, 2013:
Thaddeus in Rehabilitation

Things were progressing for Thaddeus. He had a very challenging physical therapy session this morning. He was shown how to walk using crutches. After the demonstration, he was assisted by three physical therapists to hop on the left leg and use crutches around the gym and down the hallway by the nurses' station. This was a success.

He was pretty exhausted the rest of the day. These kinds of activities require a tremendous amount of energy. After his lunch and subsequent therapy sessions—speech language, PT, and occupational therapies—he was ready to rest.

During the weekly meeting with his medical team, it was determined that he would be here another two weeks. We were exploring several options for his continued care. He might have to go to a behavioral therapy center. He would still need to continue out patient therapy, and we would make an appointment for his MCL and ACL repair on the right knee.

Thaddeus was responding normally to the medication for memory used in brain injury treatment. This had made him a little angry to realize that he was in a hospital and everyone had to take care of him. He had always been a kind and gentle patient. We prayed he would adjust to the new experience of knowing where he was with grace.

We as a family had been going through stages of grieving since the accident took place for Thaddeus. Now he was going through grief as well. First he realized that his grandparents were all gone. This was tough. Now he was realizing that his life had changed until he recovered from the brain injury. Pray for him in this grieving process. Healing can sometimes be very painful emotionally.

Asa and I had begun to research the appropriate place for Thaddeus to go in two weeks. We had some important legal matters to take care of on his behalf in September. Our ultimate goal was to get him to our home in Palm Coast for recovery.

August 29, 2013:
Thaddeus in Rehabilitation Hospital

This morning, Thaddeus had his PEG (percutaneous endoscopic gastrostomy) removed. This was a huge step in his recovery! No more tubes or lines anywhere! He was anxious to have them remove the safety belts used to keep him from falling. Once these were gone, he would be close to leaving the hospital. It was still frustrating and challenging for him.

He was able to make two tours around the nurses' station on crutches. He had another speech and language assessment to determine his attention span. There were considerable improvements. He couldn't even respond to one question when it was first done three weeks ago.

Wow, this was hard to watch. He wanted to be home, and we wanted him to be able to go home soon. We provided a familiar face and encouragement while he was here. He slept well at night, so we could leave the hospital in peace. Today we put up a calendar to show the days he had left here.

A few milestones he had to accomplish: drinking thin liquids (like water), walking by himself on crutches, minimal confusion, and no agitation. Pray for Thaddeus to find comfort and keep focused.

He told us yesterday, "I have always had a screw loose. Now it is turned sideways." We love to see his personality come through the struggles.

August 30, 2013:
Thaddeus in Rehabilitation Hospital

Today marked the sixtieth day for Thaddeus in the hospital and rehabilitation. June 29 at 11:30 p.m., life changed for all of us when a car struck Thaddeus in Lexington, Kentucky. Today we were thankful for the milestones:

Day 2—Thaddeus survived the tragic accident and was on life support

Day 7—First sign of response with moving the right hand

Day 10—Eyes opened slightly for the first time

Day 13—Thaddeus strummed the guitar placed in his hand with his right hand

Day 15—PEG and tracheostomy procedure in ICU

Day 16—Knee surgery to repair broken bone and MCL

Day 18—Thaddeus was alert and followed some verbal commands

Day 20—He was moved to progressive acute care from ICU

Day 26—Thaddeus started to talk through the trach plug

Day 30—No more oxygen, responded to commands easily

Day 32—Thaddeus was moved to the rehabilitation hospital

Day 46—First steps in the physical therapy gym between parallel bars

Day 54—First steps using a walker

Day 58—Thaddeus walked on crutches for a few steps

Day 59—PEG taken out

When we looked over the weeks of progress, it was amazing how God has blessed us. Sometimes the day to day seemed long and unchanging.

Now we were seeing Thaddeus become more mobile and start to reason and verbalize his feelings.

I would be in Palm Coast for the next few days. Asa and Jessi were going to be with Thaddeus this weekend. Thanks for praying for us.

We appreciate all of you for keeping up with Thaddeus's journey. We look forward to what lies ahead as he moves toward complete recovery one step at a time.

August 31–September 2, 2013: Thaddeus in Rehabilitation Hospital

After a couple of setbacks related to the drug therapy given to Thaddeus, he was becoming more alert again. The medicine to increase his memory caused problems and increased his agitation level. Nurses were trying to solve the concerns and gave him a drug that caused him to freak out in fear. The medication was previously used for helping him but had been stopped several days back.

He had some improvement by remembering events in his past. Thaddeus had a low understanding of what had happened and where he was. Asa was with him this weekend and had been spending a lot of time trying to help him connect some of Thaddeus's comments to reality.

My rest at home had made me feel like I needed to be in Lexington. What a challenge in thought! God says through Paul, "In whatsoever state I am therewith to be content." Okay, so I guess I never thought I would have to take this verse literally! I knew how Asa felt while he was here and I was there. This was humbling and hopeful.

I pray for the doctors and physical therapists that work with Thaddeus. He would have an appointment with the orthopedic surgeon this week to determine exactly what needed to be done with his ACL. He would see his neurosurgeon very soon for follow up on his brain injury. The team met on Tuesday morning to determine how much longer he would stay in the rehabilitation hospital.

It seemed like a lonely road for Thaddeus. As he awakened from this experience, he knew he was in a hospital but didn't know what lay ahead. We spent as much time as we could with him to help him connect. Maybe more visits would be helpful. We were happy to arrange for visits with him. He still needed pastoral visits and prayer from loving friends helping us along this journey.

September 3–5, 2013: Days 64–66 — Thaddeus in Rehabilitation Hospital

This was the long part of the journey. When Thaddeus was in ICU, his doctor told us that the traumatic brain injury recovery was similar to a marathon. It was taking both Asa and me to walk through these tough days. We appreciate all of the support.

The doctors met yesterday with the physical therapy team here at the rehabilitation hospital. They reported we were "closer to a departure date." There were several unknowns that should be cleared up over the next couple of days. Thaddeus was stabilizing with his injuries and therapies. We were learning how to help him after he left the hospital.

Tomorrow he would see the orthopedic doctor to determine what was needed to be done for his right leg. He had been non-weight-bearing on that leg since July 27. It is a challenge to use a wheelchair, walker, or crutches without being able to put any weight on the right leg. He had a calcification in his shoulder that might be contributing to the pain in his left arm.

On a lighter note, today was the dedication of the Monarch Butterfly Waystation here at the hospital. There was a presentation on the preservation of flowers and wildlife that contributed to the habitat of the monarch butterfly. My mom would have loved this event! She was partial to butterflies.

The mutation of butterflies from caterpillars to "moving flowers" parallels the healing process. Thaddeus's pain and suffering of the last few months were transforming his life into new functionality and new choices.

September 6–9, 2013: Days 67–70— Thaddeus in Rehabilitation Hospital

Thaddeus had an eventful week. He was being evaluated to leave the hospital on crutches or in a wheelchair in ten days or so. Asa requested that he be taken to the orthopedic surgeon. On Thursday we had that appointment, and now his rehabilitation had changed.

We were told that he needed no further surgeries on the right leg. He was cleared to start walking on both legs while keeping the right leg in a brace. The excitement for him was a breath of fresh air!

His physical therapist was so excited she came by to take him for a walk to see what he could do. After a stroll around the nurses' station and down the hallway and back, she was pleased! There were some new strategies in place to help him walk out of the hospital on his own! Yes!

The same day, he was taken on an outing with the physical therapy team. He went out to a live music concert with one of his friends playing in downtown Lexington. The trip was great for him, and it was so good to have him out in a normal setting. He enjoyed the music, and a friend came by to speak to him. After about an hour, we were on our way back to the hospital. It was an excellent experience. We had to give a shout-out to Heidi and Cassie! These physical therapists think outside the box.

The weekend was a slow time at the hospital since physical therapy is booked Monday through Friday. Thaddeus, Asa, and I watched football games in his room—UK won, and sadly, Florida lost. We took him out to the garden a few times, and he told us some more interesting stories. He had some friends visit, and it made his day!

Today it was great to have Alton come by to spend time with him. He always looks forward to seeing the children. We are thankful to Allison (their mom) for bringing them. Also, Thaddeus's band member from Oldman Lowdown came for a visit. Matt tuned up the PT guitar and showed Thaddeus a new song he wrote. Immediately, Thaddeus created lyrics to go with the music! We knew he had more songs that were going to come forward with time.

We are thankful for many prayers! These days were challenging for all three of us! Thaddeus continued to struggle with confusion from his brain injury. Asa would go back to Florida tomorrow. I had had a sudden allergy attack, and it was exhausting.

September 10–11, 2013:
Days 71–72—Thaddeus in Rehabilitation

Thaddeus was fully aware that he was in the hospital. The good news today was the restraints had been removed. He was not making any sporadic moves like getting up to go. Believe me, he was truly a free man right now! With realizing he was in the hospital also came the sadness that he had had a bad accident and was in the hospital. He wanted to know how long he had to stay. We awaited the results from the weekly meeting of his medical team.

I received bad news yesterday from two lawyers that there was no point to pursue a claim against the driver because they had no car insurance. It is hard to imagine that someone could be involved in an accident where a life-threatening injury took place and no one was concerned that the car was not insured. Someone help me understand.

Yesterday I called another lawyer while in Thaddeus's room. He was listening. I was describing the accident to the law office. Thaddeus corrected me and said, "I was on the curb, and the car was so close, it scared me. I jumped on my feet and fell backwards." He remembered something of the accident! It shocked both of us. He didn't know where that came from.

Today I was not at the hospital because I caught a cold—aches and all—I was keeping in touch with Thaddeus's nurse by phone. When I saw his doctor in the hallway yesterday, he said it was better to be safe than sorry. I agree.

Thankful for my Kusmi green tea (bought in France), Advil, and Juice Plus nutrition—these helped me feel better.

September 17, 2013:
Thaddeus in Rehabilitation

We are thankful for friends walking with us through this journey via social media. As I looked at the calendar, I realized that we were almost at three months of day by day. Thaddeus was recovering steadily on the plan of twelve to eighteen months of recovery. Asa and I had realized that we personally could not take care of him. The red-tape challenges were many. The medical costs were too high. The logistical support was not truly realistic. I went home for a few days so Asa and I could sort through the possibilities for Thaddeus. He loves being with us. We loved the sweet fellowship with him as he began to remember things in his life.

He had almost completed his care at Cardinal Hill Rehabilitation Hospital. His memory was better every day. He was getting better at walking distances of about 150 feet. He was beginning to climb steps. In the hospital, he had 24-7 surveillance, physical therapy, occupational therapy, psychological evaluations, and speech or language pathology. These were part of his medical plan helping him to get better. Once he left, these therapies would stop.

If we took him home with us, he would require 24-7 surveillance, months of physician follow-up, and physical or occupational therapy. He would be leaving the hospital in confusion and unstable. Because he had no insurance and Medicare was pending if we took him, he would not be able to go to an outpatient program.

We celebrate his milestones of recovery! We are thankful for God's healing of his body. Traumatic brain injury takes time. It would be an easy transition if we lived locally. Medicaid would eventually be approved and cover everything in Kentucky.

Thaddeus needed to go to a place where he could transition back to normal life, grooming, job skills, etc. I was being told there are homes that provide this environment under medical guidance. If he had insurance, there was a waiting list. If he had Medicare, he could be placed there directly from the hospital.

The place where I was staying was adequate for me to go back and forth to the hospital. The blessing of a place to stay is wonderful. This was not a good place for Thaddeus. We could take Thaddeus to Florida in his current state, but he needed medical follow-up, and I am sure you understand the high costs involved in new patient setup and home care.

Psalm 73:24–26 (ESV) says, "You will guide me with your counsel . . . whom have I in heaven but you? And there is nothing on earth that I desire besides you. My flesh and my heart may fail, but God is the strength of my heart and my portion forever."

September 18, 2013:
Thaddeus in Rehabilitation Hospital

In physical therapy, Thaddeus was able to climb two flights of stairs. He was making such great progress with his walking and stability. He still needed supervision when walking (and step climbing). He was exhausted after a few minutes of walking.

He had more ability to carry on a normal conversation for a longer period of time. The side effects of his brain injury included something called perseveration. This meant he kept repeating something over and over without knowing he was repeating. A few weeks ago, the subjects were related to be in restraints. Thaddeus still could perseverate on something all day long about getting out of the hospital.

We would have a meeting with the care manager and Thaddeus's doctor specialized in rehabilitation medicine. They would put together a plan for his discharge from the hospital. We needed prayer in every direction!

Today I was finally able to retrieve Thaddeus's personal effects from the accident. He had his cell phone, hat, shoes, and wallet. It was too sad for him to look at the broken neck of the guitar.

I had a special surprise visit with my friend Denise from AT&T. How cool was that!

Posted on Facebook:
Thaddeus Greear
September 17, 2013
head leg and arm feeling rehabbed

September 19–20, 2013:
Days 80–81—Thaddeus in Rehabilitation

We are thankful for prayers. The days of struggle and drama seemed to melt into peace yesterday afternoon. We were seeing the light at the end of this tunnel for Thaddeus. He sent his first text message from his phone yesterday. I was finally able to get his personal belongings from the police department.

Yesterday he spoke with the client relations representative from the NeuroRestorative Residential program in Lexington. This is a home where traumatic-brain-injury patients go for ongoing therapies and transition to independent living with a nursing staff and a rehabilitation doctor on call. They have a teaching kitchen as well as a music recording studio with skilled musicians working with the patients. His acceptance into the program required approval of his pending Medicaid and a brain waiver issued by the state. We were told a bed might be available next week.

Thaddeus and I went out to dinner last night. The rehabilitation center gave him a day pass (four hours) for me to take him out of the center. We invited his children to join us at Ramsey's for dinner. Thaddeus ordered a burger with bacon and cheese—I think he was happy not to have hospital food. He still had some concerns in public.

He enjoyed spending time with Holton. It is truly a blessing to see him doing so well.

September 24, 2013: Day 85—Thaddeus in the Rehabilitation Hospital

T haddeus continued to make progress physically in his rehabilitation at Cardinal Hill. We heard this morning that he had been approved for the Emergency Brain Injury Waiver list, and this stepped many things forward for his continued care.

Today we were working on setting up appointments with medical doctors after his departure from the hospital. He would have some post-injury psychological evaluations in the next few days. His trauma was affecting his anxiety. This can be stressful for all of us at times. Pray we could get him to the right doctors.

In all things, God "delivers and rescues; He works signs and wonders in heaven and on earth" (Dan. 6:27). His hand upon Thaddeus is being demonstrated live and direct for these truths.

My abilities to cope with all the obstacles had challenged me to the core. It is clear that in my own strength, I would have walked away before today. The desperation moments and exasperation moments had always been followed by a strong word from the Lord to keep on going. Any journey of this nature is difficult, and it takes a good support network to handle this on earth. We are thankful for the support!

We were submitting paperwork for the scholarship program for Brooks Rehabilitation Center in Jacksonville, Florida. Thaddeus would go on a waiting list for January or February. There were three ahead of him, and they are providing funding for one person per month.

Friday afternoon, Thaddeus and I visited the NeuroRestorative program and were quite impressed. We were on track for the day program at the Lexington Program and, hopefully, the NeuroRestorative Home. The departure date from Cardinal Hill was pending. Thaddeus was anxious to leave the hospital. I am thankful he knew where he was and wanted to leave.

September 29–30, 2013:
Thaddeus in Rehabilitation Hospital

Wow! Three months had come and gone for Thaddeus since his tragic accident. He was moving forward toward the NeuroRestorative Home in Kentucky. He received the Acquired Brain Injury waiver on Wednesday. We were processing paperwork to get him transferred from the rehabilitation hospital.

Asa and I toured the facility and a home here in Lexington on Friday. There are many important therapies, including physical therapy, occupational therapy, speech-language pathology, music therapy, art therapy, group therapies, and reintegration to normal living activities. We prayed his transition into the program went well.

Jeremiah and Chelsi arrived on Sunday! It had been a sweet reunion for Thaddeus with his brother. They had had lots of laughs, and it had been fun to see Thaddeus so excited.

On Monday, Thaddeus had a visit with his neurosurgeon at University of Kentucky Medical Clinic. She said he had "graduated" from needing her services any longer. He told her he didn't like to be "held captive." She told him he was being "held in love" and to enjoy it. (Go, Doctor!)

Thaddeus walked wherever he needed to go now. We had to secure his stability. His wheelchair had been parked in the room for a few days now. He remembered a lot of what happened the day before. When asked in the afternoon, he remembered most of the morning events. He recognized his lapses of memory and even apologized to us when he made a mistake. These were positive steps toward recovery.

The hardest thing about life for Thaddeus was understanding how and why he got to the hospital. He didn't understand many things about this experience, and it frustrated him, causing anxiety. He could switch from laughter to sadness to anger to harsh words to sweet friendliness in a matter of seconds. This is normal brain-injury-recovery behavior. Pray for all of us in these days.

October 7, 2013:
Thaddeus in Rehabilitation Hospital

Thaddeus was enjoying family today! Holton and Alton were on fall break from school, so they hung out with Daddy all day. Jeremiah and Chelsi brought him breakfast. His birthday week was off to a great start!

This morning, a jury of six and the judge awarded me guardianship for Thaddeus. I told him I was his new guardian angel. He had already given permission. Since the lawyers, the hospital staff, the court-appointed psychologist, Thaddeus, and I were all in agreement, I didn't have to testify. I appreciated Thaddeus's lawyer in his opening statement, "Your positive response will be an act of love."

This step allowed me to process his Medicare and disability paperwork and help him get into the programs that would help him improve.

Tomorrow I would meet with a new lawyer to assist in expediting the paperwork red tape. There were still several steps to be taken before he could get into the NeuroRestorative program in Louisville or Lexington. There are beds available in both programs. He could not move until the Medicare and disability process was complete.

I have all three of my children and all grandchildren in the same state. What a blessing! We continued to press forward in all this. Your prayers and support keep us going.

On October 10, Thaddeus posted on Facebook:

> Thaddeus here. Thanks to everyone for the birthday wishes. Healing in my head and love in my heart for all.

October 15, 2013:
Thaddeus in the Rehabilitation Hospital

We are thankful for all who have kept us in their prayers and thoughts! Traumatic brain injury has a long recovery period. In Thaddeus's case, it will take thirteen more months to see full recovery. I am including here some of the things we are dealing with as Thaddeus understands his limitations:

- **A Healthy Brain**

  To understand what happens when the brain is injured, it is important to realize what a healthy brain is made of and what it does. The brain is enclosed inside the skull. The skull acts as a protective covering for the soft brain. The brain is made of neurons (nerve cells). The neurons form tracts that route throughout the brain. These nerve tracts carry messages to various parts of the brain. The brain uses these messages to perform functions. The functions include our coordinating our body's systems, such as breathing, heart rate, body temperature, and metabolism; thought processing; body movements; personality; behavior; and the senses, such as vision, hearing, taste, smell, and touch. Each part of the brain serves a specific function and links with other parts of the brain to form more complex functions. All parts of the brain need to be working well in order for the brain to work well. Even "minor" or "mild" injuries to the brain can significantly disrupt the brain's ability to function.

- **An Injured Brain**

  When a brain injury occurs, the functions of the neurons, nerve tracts, or sections of the brain can be affected. If the neurons and nerve tracts are affected, they can be unable or have difficulty carrying the messages that tell the brain what to do. This can change the way a person thinks, acts, feels, and moves the body. Brain injury can also change the complex internal functions of the body, such as regulating body temperature; blood pressure; bowel and bladder control. These changes can be temporary or permanent. They may cause impairment or a complete inability to perform a function.

Thaddeus was progressing in his physical and occupational therapy. The levels of achievement included making appointments with the nurse for medications, going to meals on his own, and interviewing the staff to understand their jobs. He was able to fully shower, shave, and dress himself with minimal assistance. The monotony of being in a hospital room with little activity was challenging.

Today (October 15, 2013), his case was reopened for Social Security Disability. With many months of working on these processes, we saw light at the end of the red-tape tunnel. Pray for those who would evaluate Thaddeus's injury and make the decision to approve his disability. He would be able to go into the NeuroRestorative program upon approval.

October 16, 2013

Back in Kentucky. Taking Thaddeus to see his orthopedic surgeon tomorrow. Pray for him to find peace.

October 23, 2013: Day 116—
Thaddeus in the Rehabilitation Hospital:
Countdown to Departure

The daily updates had become weekly updates since Thaddeus was making such great progress. He was able to get a new brace for his right leg yesterday. This one was lightweight and gave him more stability.

The DonJoy representative met with us personally yesterday morning. Amazing how much you can get done quickly by negotiating with the company. I was able get a two- to three-week waiting period turned into next-day service. Whew!

We were still waiting for the decisions for Thaddeus's medical benefits to process. We were happy he was going to be able to go to the NeuroRestorative Program. Meanwhile, we had a game of "hurry up and wait" with the red-tape processes. The placement was guaranteed once everything was approved.

On Monday we made a decision to go ahead and take Thaddeus out of the hospital. He was going to be going into therapy at University of Louisville Medical Center starting Tuesday of next week. He had a few more days of intense physical therapies at Cardinal Hill. We are very thankful for the physical therapy and occupational therapy at Cardinal Hill.

Changes are challenging for Thaddeus. Pray for him in the process.

Thaddeus had been struggling with some negativity for several weeks. I put a post on Facebook, asking for prayer, and it surprised him. It was tough for him to be in the hospital, realize that his life had completely changed, and he had many months to go before he would recover. He responded to me with love, and we are now able to talk about his feelings and expressions more openly. Each day has a different challenge.

From the beginning, Thaddeus had said, "I just want to be with my mom and dad to learn again the things they taught me." Well, we were ready to begin the next phase of the journey as Thaddeus went home on my birthday, October 25.

October 25, 2013:
Day 1 in Louisville, Kentucky

We were staying in a home sponsored by the Beechmont Baptist Church. The generosity of the church members is wonderful. They have an old-style Kentucky home in a nice older neighborhood behind Churchill Downs.

We had been staying near the Cardinal Hill Rehabilitation Hospital in Lexington, Kentucky, off Alexandria Drive. The convenience of the apartment outweighed the tough shape we found ourselves staying in. Changing neighborhoods can present unique challenges to churches.

I left Lexington with hesitation last week to look at this house. My heart just wanted to go home. Thaddeus needed help for a few more weeks until he could get into full-time NeuroRestorative programs. The house would give us a place to rest and be more comfortable. I would drive him back and forth to the University of Louisville for therapy.

In every step of this journey, I feel as though I have lead feet walking to the next step. Staying in a hotel in the beginning was familiar but not practical. It was tough to transition to the apartment. For three months, I had found a way to settle some so that I did more than just go to the hospital. As I was beginning to settle, this door opened for us in Louisville.

Thaddeus would get better outpatient care here. The programs he would be a part of set trends for the entire state. When he got approved for Social Security Disability, I could get him into the NeuroRestorative program on his Acquired Brain Injury waiver. Full coverage would be available for him.

Emotionally, I was a wreck. I would tear up at a moment's notice. My heart was weary from the drama of the last four months. My body was physically upset with wrong nutrition, no regular exercise, and discomfort becoming a way of life.

Only God can help me through each and every day. I look to him when I am waking up and lying down to sleep. He gives me rest and helps me to keep on. When the table is full of challenging things, I have to give everything to him and go to bed. Then he opens the door for my next step.

Tomorrow I would celebrate my first birthday without my mama. The last one I spent at her house. I felt compelled to spend my birthday with my mom last year. On December 23, I knew why. God wanted me to have that moment with her however short it was. He gives us so many blessings in the most unusual ways. Today I was thankful to have had that day with her.

Asa would come in from Palm Coast tonight, and tomorrow we would take Thaddeus home from the hospital for the second time in his life. The days ahead were open for new challenges. He was walking, talking, and taking care of his own shower and toilet needs. He was able to help out around the house some.

In the mornings, he forgot some things but overall was doing quite well!

October 29, 2013

Asa was here with me. Wow, how much that calmed my heart and weary mind! He was able to join us for Friday-morning departure from the hospital in Lexington. He planned to stay a few weeks with us to get settled into the house.

We are thankful for the transitional apartment I stayed in near Cardinal Hill Hospital. It was a gracious gift that was functional. I moved near Thaddeus's therapy in Louisville the day before he left the hospital.

We had everything we needed in a comfortable home for the next few months of stay in Kentucky. The home is a ministry of a wonderful group of people. The old-style Louisville home has three stories and is fully furnished. We only had to move in with suitcases! They had opened their hearts and arms for Coco Chanel to stay with her family. She has a fenced-in yard to explore and a comfy spot at the bottom of the staircase.

Thaddeus was doing very well at "home." He had settled in well and even helped out. We were still waiting on Social Security Disability and Medicaid to be approved for Thaddeus to cover his medical costs. Right now we were paying out of our pockets on any medical care he needed. In the grand scheme of things, we believed this would be approved soon.

In everything, we give thanks! I had a great birthday weekend. Jessi and her family spent the weekend with us. Ary and Juliette had fun going up and down the stairs. Alton was able to spend the first few days with his daddy home from the hospital. He was happy Mimi had gotten the Internet installed so he could keep up with his video games.

We had come a long way in this journey and looked forward to the next transition—going home to Florida in a few months! In the meantime, we would take Thaddeus to University of Louisville tomorrow for his evaluations for physical therapy, occupational therapy, and speech-language pathology.

Jessi was very close to her due date for baby number 3—Aiden. He was scheduled to arrive in Campbellsville on November 25. If this baby was like the two girls, we could see him anytime after this week. Arya and Juliette were both three weeks early.

God had planted us near her for a few months while Thaddeus continued his treatments and healing. God is good.

Thaddeus updated his new Facebook page:

October 30, 2013

i didn't think that I had that many memories to forget with a brain injury. Shoot

November 3, 2013

Thaddeus was progressing in his therapy. He was able to stop taking one medication and had settled well into our new temporary home in Louisville. Therapy was hard work, and the time change had confused him somewhat. All in all, we were very pleased with the positive changes.

Thaddeus and I had become partners in pumpkin pie making. He mixed the filling, and I put it in the oven to bake. He played his guitar daily and was getting better each time.

Thaddeus on Day 6 at "home." One picture is worth a thousand words. — with Thaddeus Greear.

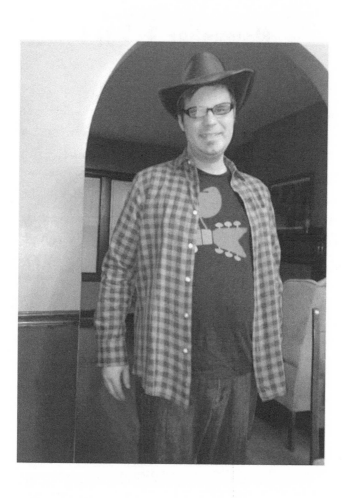

November 8, 2013

Mission accomplished! By the grace of God, I had a PERK (only he knows what that stands for) from SSA. Next Wednesday they would call with a number! That magic number got his NeuroRestorative treatment.

At this time, we had been placed on deferment status until February 1 for Social Security Disability. This impacted Thaddeus's long-term care. We know God is bigger than government programs and medical-assistance decision makers. I prayed we could find insurance coverage for Thaddeus to continue his care. I would be working on getting him temporary Medicaid tomorrow. Thanks for keeping up with us. Progress was slow. The doctor support was needed for disability, and this was the reason for his deferment. Only God.

November 10, 2013: Thaddeus Update

It had been four and a half months since Thaddeus was walking across an intersection and hit by a car in Lexington, Kentucky. We had seen him come a long way from the ER to neurosurgical ICU to acute care to rehabilitation care and out to wait for entry into the NeuroRestorative program.

Today Thaddeus and I went to church together. He was impressed by the pastor at Beechmont Baptist Church and remembered the sermons. Today we heard a message on courage. Interesting how God always works through his Word. I was just studying Daniel 11:18–21 on Friday afternoon while waiting in the Social Security office to assure Thaddeus's paperwork was entered into the system.

God's message to Daniel was for different reasons than mine. It was a timely moment: "He said, 'O man of high esteem, do not be afraid. Peace be with you; take courage and be courageous!' Now as soon as he spoke to me, I received strength and said, 'May my lord speak, for you have strengthened me.'"

After telling me they couldn't do anything for me and my persistence in courage, Danielle (my SSA admin) had a change of heart. She told me to wait and they would call me by name to another office to fill out paperwork. Juanita (wearing an Origami Owl Locket) processed Thaddeus's "presumptive" Medicaid coverage retroactive to August. Exhausted, I was relieved and, believe it or not, angry—not sure where that anger came from. I thanked the Lord for blessing.

Our precious friend, Joni Cracraft, sat with Thaddeus at Bob Evans while I negotiated with the Social Security Administration. Joni and Carlos have stood by us all the way.

Swirls of emotion and challenge keep us on our toes. Thaddeus was struggling with the visit tomorrow with the NeuroRestorative home and facility. I was also challenged with releasing him to yet another unknown. We just need your prayers.

Asa was holding everything together in Palm Coast in Palm Coast. His ministry was thriving under these circumstances. Sometimes I just felt Thaddeus and I were alone walking this journey. We are surrounded by many prayers and loving words to us via e-mail, text, and Facebook. God is always walking with us each day.

November 12:
Case Manager for Traumatic
Brain Injury Medicaid Waiver

We had appointments with the vision specialist, neuropsychiatrist, and physiatrist!

November 20, 2013 Thaddeus update

Our journey continues and new days are ahead. As things fall into place we know that God is orchestrating everything. Yesterday Thaddeus was introduced to his new Physiatrist. The neuro rehabilitation doctor will take care of Thaddeus' medical needs while he is in the Neuro Restorative program. We have many things to be thankful for:

Thaddeus survived a tragic accident as a pedestrian hit by a car on June 29
Thaddeus woke up from a coma on July 15
Thaddeus was transferred to Cardinal Hill Rehabilitation Hospital on July 31
"Heart of Gold" Benefit Concert was held for Thaddeus by his precious friends organized by Sherri McGee August 2
Thaddeus walked for the first time on August 15
Thaddeus was able to go on an outing from the hospital on August 16
Jeremiah turned 35 on August 22
Thaddeus walked unassisted on September 5
Thaddeus left Cardinal Hill Rehabilitation Hospital October 25
Jeremiah and Chelsi moved to Tallahassee October 28

Jessi and Ryan welcomed Aiden Alexandre into the world on November 15
Thaddeus was approved to receive Community Rehabilitation at the
NeuroRestorative Center starting on November 21, 2013

Each milestone of the journey with Thaddeus has been a blessing.
Our family enters this Thanksgiving season thankful for many things!

November 26, 2013

We were thankful that Asa was returning to Kentucky today to prepare for Thanksgiving. We were thankful Jessi and Ryan and family would join us for Thanksgiving dinner. We were thankful that Jeremiah and Chelsi were settling well into their new home in Tallahassee! We were thankful for a church that had allowed us to rent this lovely home full of grace and charm.

Thaddeus was adjusting to his therapies at the NeuroRestorative Community Rehabilitation Center. Today was his fourth day to go. It was challenging for him to take this step. Each day, we had motivation moments to get him started.

Today we listened to a precious song my mom (in heaven now) used to sing to me. Nat King Cole was one of her and Daddy's favorite artists. We listened to "Smile."

It made me cry, and Thaddeus listened carefully. It was a tender moment before he got out of the car for the day.

It is not easy to accept that he has a traumatic brain injury. It is not easy to be away from home for so long. It is not easy to create a home away from home. It is not easy to know what lies ahead. It is not easy to walk forward with lead feet. God is sufficient to cover our needs.

Baby Aiden is adorable! He is the sweetest little fella and such a blessing to our family. Jessi and Ryan and the girls were adjusting very well. I am so thankful for this new life and precious gift to our family!

Pray for Thaddeus as he would enter the house for NeuroRestorative on Monday, December 2. It was a tough transition. He would be there on a trial basis. That was my commitment to him. We would have a thirty meeting on December 21 to discuss his progress and goals for the program. He was working with his therapists to set these goals now. We had full medical coverage until February 1 for him to participate.

There were still many unknowns. I would change my Facebook photo today to the Brain Injury Awareness Ribbon. This journey is a challenge, and we are thankful for those who walk with us forward each day!

December 10, 2013

Christmas was around the corner, and we prepared to celebrate Christ's birth. Thaddeus had finished his first week in the residence at NeuroRestorative Community Rehabilitation. God is faithful. Thaddeus knew that this step was important for him to be able to get back to life on his own. It was a tough transition. We had made a commitment to keep moving forward for his benefit even if it was awkward.

Personally, I was exhausted after several weeks of the intensity of transition from rehabilitation hospital to outpatient therapy to NeuroRestorative and then to the NR residence. Today I was happy to be in Palm Coast with Asa, enjoying my home and the warm Florida weather. This was a special joy in the journey.

Here are other things we had enjoyed over the past two weeks:

- Had Thaddeus at home—be able to pray with him and love on him every day
- Celebrated with Jessi's family during Thanksgiving
- Heard Thaddeus's heart on how God is working in his life
- Got to know the pastor and his wife at Beechmont Baptist Church

Each step of the journey comes with a challenge of transition. We had come to a point where there were fewer unknowns. We know the trials of brain injury are real. We knew Thaddeus had months of therapies ahead of him to become independent. He has good days and bad days. He remembers more every day.

Here's an example: When we were in France, I bought Thaddeus an Arabic teapot. It was a longstanding request from him. Before the injury, he loved to brew Chinese green tea buds and make strong Arabic tea. This was something he did while living in West Africa. The first of December, I showed him the teapot as well as the small tea glasses used when drinking the hot tea. He didn't understand anything about the teapot, glasses, or brewing tea.

Then while visiting with him last Wednesday (December 4), we went to a Middle Eastern restaurant to eat dinner. At the restaurant, he talked to me in great detail about making tea in Africa. I told him about the teapot and the glasses that I bought for him from France. He was thrilled! He asked where the teapot was. I told him it was at the guesthouse and that I would bring it to him when I got back. (Smile.)

Little by little, new pathways were being created to old memories. We were at five and half months into this journey. God is working miracles in Thaddeus's life. His healing path was a third of the way complete, by medical calculations.

December 18, 2013: NeuroRestorative Individual Development Team Meeting

After introductions all around and sharing that we were meeting to discuss Thaddeus's first month at NR, progress, hopes and planning, Thaddeus shared the following:

- I am working hard to get better.
- I want to get my life back.
- I am grateful to this group for all the help I'm receiving.
- My new glasses are great (smiling, telling about his visit to Dr. Weinberg, showing the glasses he is wearing and expressing that new glasses are on order).
- My knee pain is now about a six, which is down from an eight when it was first hit.

Counseling shared these:

- She and Thaddeus talked about the IDT before arriving, discussing his thoughts or hopes.
- Thaddeus was doing extremely well, praise and encouragement shared.
- He was running into anxiety and mental fatigue, which was expected at this point in recovery.
- She was working with his team to take needed breaks during care.

- She validated the immense stress of all the changes over the past weeks, moving to Louisville, beginning programming, moving into residential setting, etc.
- She provided feedback about managing personal-space issues and the involvement of visual challenges, Thaddeus having expressed the feeling of being too close at times when speaking to others.
- Recent changes and new events had increased his anxiety level and decreased his energy level—not unexpected.
- Thaddeus's emotional energy would increase as his anxiety decreased, as things became more familiar.
- She validated that this was not a big growth period, but more for learning, structure.
- She discussed that this ABI or accident happens to a whole family.
- She gave encouragement to Thaddeus to be in things on which he'd like to work and things to discuss.

Occupational Therapy Assistant, with an OTA student observing, shared these:

- She praised Thaddeus for his determination and hard work.
- They'd been working on fine motor or grasping tasks.
- Thaddeus had finished tasks without pain or tingling.
- They were practicing fine motor exercises, touching left thumb to each individual left finger (Thaddeus demonstrating as she spoke).
- She offered to take Thaddeus for a haircut as group discussed finances or planning.
- They discussed plans for a trip to have ID made, planning for the coming Friday, if possible.

Speech Language Pathologist shared these:

- After her group discussion of hearing concerns, she would speak with nursing RE: audiologist referral.
- She praised Thaddeus for making such strong progress.
- She noted STM, organizational, and two- to three-step sequencing struggles.
- They focused on language, skills, and processing in his care or planning.
- They were working on reasoning tasks, searching recipes on the computer: navigating the Internet (using mouse and working up to keyboard), finding the recipes, writing lists for the grocery trip, and plans to implement these recipes into cooking.
- She had seen Thaddeus demonstrate such determination and positive forward movement in his therapy.
- They were working on speech inflection and the social impact involved.

Occuptional Therapist shared the following:

- She gave praise to Thaddeus for his determination and positive spirit.
- She worked with him to do typing for fine-motor movement, specifically of the left hand.
- Typing upset Thaddeus as it reminded him of songwriting.
- Attempts to play the guitar upset Thaddeus as they were disappointing
- They went to the music store together, and Thaddeus screened a guitar instruction book for her as she has always desired to play (Thaddeus smiling).
- She pointed out that the music room at NR might be intimidating due to multiple people there as well as them already able to play (Thaddeus nodding).

- Thaddeus was agreeable to playing music or guitar with one person at a time at his home (Thaddeus nodding and with verbal agreement).
- Thaddeus had expressed wanting to grow his hair longer as it had been before.
- He discussed plans for trip to get a haircut, specifically with another occupational therapy assistant.
- She would contact U of L PT for exercises as he attended PT with them regularly (later e-mail sent that she had already initiated contact).
- She expressed possibility of a support group for mother or family.
- There were specifics of needed info for an ID card (cost was twenty dollars, needed SS card and proof of address).
- There was the possibility of mother or family attending support group (follow up e-mail sent later from ABI case manager with support group info).

Internal Case Manager shared the following:

- Validation and immense praise for Thaddeus' positive adjustment to so many changes.
- She reviewed with Thaddeus his desires (music, haircut, PT, etc.) throughout the meeting.
- Music therapist or therapy was not likely to be contracted by NR, focusing on what the program did offer, especially R/T Thaddeus.
- Notation of upcoming appointments, discussion of medical needs or scheduling.
- Consents were discussed, confirming contact info.

Lydia (Thaddeus's mother) shared the following:

- Desire for Thaddeus to have a dental visit.
- Update of vision care visit, including new glasses to be ready by January 8, 2014.
- Vacation dates for Thaddeus to go to Florida with his parents: Sunday, December 22 to Wednesday, January 1, 2014.
- Scheduled MD visit to Neuropsychiatrist on Thursday, January 2 at 1:20 p.m., with plans to return to programming after that.
- Thaddeus's spacial concerns R/T vision needs.
- Inquired about referral for ENT or audiologist for hearing challenges or possible deficits (group discussion, with audiologist referral TBA).
- Concern that Thaddeus's trust issues might be keeping him from connecting with the musician that visits twice weekly.
- Inquiry about possibility of a music therapist or U of L music therapy students coming to NR.
- Wanted to see PT exercises in his daily program, noting that the U of L PT worked wonderfully with him, and he couldn't maintain the growth without daily exercises.
- Not seeing or hearing global progress for Thaddeus.
- Today was "point zero" and a move forward and to see things progress.
- Thaddeus was "mad at her" for putting him into residential housing.
- Thaddeus has always been a fast learner.
- Grooming is a big issue in their family.
- Concerned that he was not brushing his teeth or trimming or washing his beard.
- Felt he needed to work on his intonation to differentiate emotions in conversations.
- It is a double-edged sword—referring to the interpersonal situation with his ex-wife and children.

Thaddeus shared these:

- Thanks to all on his team.
- Demonstration of one of his PT exercises (attempt to crumple a paper using one hand only).
- Walking was getting stronger and steadier.
- Felt it was his fault that walker hit his knee several days ago (all verified not his fault).
- He was working on differentiating conversations around him, feeling it was improving.
- That his music dream "is in there!"
- He had to shower at the house every morning.
- He wanted to grow his beard and keep it groomed.
- He wanted his hair to be longer, like it was before (showing photos to the group).
- He had seventeen dollars hidden in his room and an insurance card as he was trying to be independent as he was before.
- He would like to go out for a haircut.
- He asked his mother for money about every two weeks and wanted to learn to budget it himself.
- Quoting lyrics to a song about money or means, expressed that he felt he could manage with twenty dollars per week.
- Expressed confidence in his U of L PT.
- Doesn't like being called brain injured.

After each attendee had a chance to share, the entire group discussed music hopes or plans, and Thaddeus seemed cautiously optimistic about playing a bit with one person at his house. I reminded him how very early in his recovery this really was, which his whole therapy team chimed in to support, all of us offering encouragement and support. Discussion ensued about money or budgeting. With his mother as his guardian and Thaddeus adamant about managing his own money, the team offered a plan to assist him to budget for such events as haircut, spontaneous outings, such as McDonald's visit. Plans were confirmed to attempt to obtain ID this Friday, thanks to Samantha for planning to transport or accompany.

Visit concluded with a review, thanks shared all around, and the echoed sentiment of what a joy it is to work with Thaddeus, and hope resounding for his progress.

December 29, 2013: Thaddeus Update

We had a wonderful Christmas! Thaddeus was able to travel by car from Louisville to Palm Coast on Sunday, December 22. We were all a little weary from traveling, but it was wonderful to have him here for Christmas. We are thankful for loving support during this holiday season.

Thaddeus was with us to celebrate two Christmases—one with Jessi and Ryan and family. We spent December 23 through Christmas Day with Jeremiah and Chelsi. God had given us much this year.

One year ago today, we had a sweet graveside service on the chilly Patton Cemetery Hill for my mom. She spent her second Christmas in heaven this year. Wow, it has been tough to get through the holidays without her.

Here is a recap of our blessings for 2013: Thaddeus is alive and moving forward in his therapies. We are thankful he can walk and care for himself. He has received appropriate financial support to cover his medical expenses. He is getting stronger and remembering more every day.

Aiden Alexandre! Jessi, Ryan, Ary, and Juliette are enjoying their new addition. He is a special blessing to all of us! He was almost six weeks old. What a sweet baby! He is a special blessing to all of us! Mama and baby are doing great!

Jeremiah and Chelsi moved to Tallahassee! We are so happy to have them nearer to home. Jeremiah works for Firestone, and Chelsi works with an educational program from FSU. Their schnauzers, Anabel and Molly, are cute as can be. We were so happy to have them with us through Christmas Day.

St. Johns River Baptist Association! Churches are blessed by Asa's loving care and heart for ministry leaders. We have been in Florida for seven years now. Loving the weather and trying to find time for fun!

I retired early from AT&T in May and then prepared for our great adventure to France. Alton, Thaddeus's son, was able to go with us for the first time. What a fun trip! Since our return from France, I have been staying between Palm Coast and Kentucky to help Thaddeus, enjoying the blessings of my family being near.

We pray 2014 is peaceful and productive. Thaddeus had several doctor appointments in January. He would begin vision therapy with a specialist. His stay in the NeuroRestorative residential program is a challenge. We were not sure how long he would stay before we took him home. We had another Social Security date of February 1. This would determine how long he would remain.

January 7, 2014

Bonne année! Happy New Year! We were enjoying the wishes of friends from around the world as we finished our first week of 2014. Thaddeus continued to tell me every day, "I just want to be with my family." We are working toward that goal day by day.

Today, Thaddeus returned to the NeuroRestorative residence and program after a great seventeen-day break! Thaddeus and I discussed his return to the center when we were within a few blocks. I told him, "It is the right thing to do." He agreed with me, "It is the right thing to do."

Then I went to do some errands. I left a bag of VIA coffee (he drank this every morning because the residence only bought decaf) in the bag on the floor at Starbucks. I went to an appointment with music therapy at University of Louisville and parked beautifully on the curb. I headed back to the house and then remembered the coffee was missing. I went to finish the errands and picked him up.

The staff was amazed to see his progress while he was away with us! Comments from everyone reflected how well he was walking, talking, and his general well-being. He was excited to get a library card during his occupational therapy. I asked if he got some books. He said, "No, you have to return them."

We went out to Chili's and enjoyed a great meal. He settled into the house and I left. Then I broke down. Yes, it is the right thing to do, but these are the hardest things I have ever done in my life.

January 21, 2014

Deep in the cold and snow of Louisville, Kentucky, Thaddeus and I enjoyed a few days together. Thaddeus had had several appointments with doctors and continuing therapies. He was fitted for a new pair of glasses, which included prisms and correction for his eyes. After waiting for approvals, he received the glasses last Friday.

Within a few days, he was seeing better. It was fun when he spontaneously started reading the road signs to me in the car. This was a first! The neuro-optometrist would begin therapy for Thaddeus next week. Thaddeus was given a thorough testing for different issues related to the impact of his head injury on his eyes.

The nerves in the eye impact the entire body. In spite of doctors and therapists discouraging us from getting his vision checked by a specialist, we learned that this is necessary as soon as a TBI patient wakes up from the coma. It took me three months to convince someone to get us an appointment. He would undergo therapy or treatment for *binocular vision conditions*, such as *amblyopia or lazy eye, convergence insufficiency* (near vision disorder), *diplopia* (double vision), *lack of stereopsis* (two-eyed depth perception), and *strabismus* (cross-eyed, wandering eye, eye turns, etc.).

Our visit with the ear, nose, and throat specialist was cancelled due to the snowstorm. We were following up on his nose fractures and auditory concerns. Thaddeus and I agree that we were tired of seeing so many doctors. Yet each one brought a special aspect to his healing process. The physiatrist followed his overall health.

He had an amazing physical therapist who was helping correct his gait, arm movements, and reconnection of the left side of his body. He saw her twice per week at the University of Louisville. His new glasses helped a lot!

At NeuroRestorative, we were pleased with the positive changes to his therapy team. After the meeting with the team in December, he was given a new occupational therapist, who was a musician and could connect with Thaddeus on music.

At the residence, it was still difficult for Thaddeus to be comfortable. Yesterday he told me that he was told, "This house is as much mine as it is the others." This is a milestone that he had a hard time accomplishing because one TBI patient was controlling everything in the home.

We pray for Thaddeus in his adjustments. I was able to go home more often due to his transition to the residence. We wanted Thaddeus to come home to Florida for a few months as soon as he was able. He wanted to be able to get a job and save money to move back to his life in Lexington. The journey continued.

January 30, 2014

We are rejoicing in every positive step Thaddeus takes in his journey toward recovery. It is hard to believe he was hit seven months ago. He works hard in occupational therapy plus physical therapy and wants so much to have his life back. I just wish he knew how many sideline cheerleaders were praying and supporting him.

Today I took him to his doctor appointments, and it was precious to sit and drink coffee with him knowing he is getting better every day. We have more normal conversations. He loves his children and misses them so much. Living in the NeuroRestorative house was still very hard for him. Today he told me that his change was missing from the dresser in his room. He said, "The saddest part is that I am afraid to talk about it to someone."

Tomorrow he would begin a long weekend at our home away from home in Louisville. We were looking forward to the time together. He wanted to shave his beard, so we'd go find a barber to help him out.

February 19, 2014

"The name of the Lord is a strong tower; the righteous run to it and are safe" (Prov. 18:10).

The Lord is our strong tower—we run to it. Today I returned to Louisville to get Thaddeus to his ENT appointment tomorrow. As usual, prior to my arrival and upon arrival, there were concerns. Normally I don't count on trouble, yet the pattern had emerged.

I had a smooth flight (delayed but not bad) last night and watched God's hand carried me back to Thaddeus. Prior to departure, I received two phone calls. The first caller informed me that Thaddeus's Medicaid was inactive. This meant he might not have any coverage until the disability was confirmed. The next call was to say that he would no longer have appointments for physical therapy because he had no insurance coverage. His prescriptions could not be filled at this time because he had no Medicaid. His disability was under review, and they needed more documentation. So if there are any SSI-Medicaid specialists out there who have a way around things, I am all ears!

We had to postpone his appointment until next month. Tomorrow I would be going back to the Social Security office to find out what was going on. Meanwhile, I was looking into ObamaCare, which could start on April 1 even if we were approved. But he had no income because he has a head injury.

Asa and I would have the pleasure of spending the entire weekend with Thaddeus. I looked forward to seeing him tomorrow. I'd send out an update then.

Friday, February 21, 2014

Today I woke up at 6:30 a.m. and stumbled down the stairs to the kitchen. Inside a large black toolbox were the prepackaged packets of medications for Thaddeus given to me by the NeuroRestorative rehabilitation program nursing staff. When I picked up Thaddeus on Thursday, I signed a form stating that I received the medications. I looked over the form to assure the count for the drugs was correct.

At 6:30 a.m., I saw that Thaddeus's dosage of Zyprexa had been increased by 2.5 mg. He had two packets of Zyprexa. The total dosage was 12 mg. Included in the boxes were two packets of Zyprexa for 10 mg and 2.5 mg. The dosage had increased from February 4 when I dropped him off at the NR facility before my departure. This medication is given to Thaddeus as a mood stabilizer to assist him in combating the mood swings resulting from his bipolar disorder.

Last night, Thaddeus was exhibiting a change in his personality. He was worried about people thinking he was gay. He was upset about his underwear not being clean. When I tried to hug him or console him, he became angry and agitated that I had tried to touch him. This morning he was again agitated and upset that I had tried to hug him.

Immediately I contacted the neuropsychiatrist office and also spoke with Thaddeus's physiatrist. I left a message for someone in the records department at Dr. office to contact me about the notes on Thaddeus's chart.

The physiatrist's assistant sent me a text with two scripts that had been received from neurospsychiatrist's office. One was a copy of the handwritten script I had given them after Thaddeus's first visit. The second was an e-form sent on January 30.

Several text messages went back and forth with me insisting that the doctor call me. She suggested that I e-mail him and he would respond back to me. I composed an e-mail with my concern.

I spoke immediately with nursing upon arrival at the NR facility. The nursing staff showed me the prescription documents. I asked for the paper I had signed when returning his medications on February 4. They said it was in the file and did not look for it. I told them not to give him any more of the added dosage of Zyprexa until we were able to confirm with the doctor.

I received a reply from the physiatrist. He shared my concern and agreed on the logic behind the increase. He said he would investigate. He contacted nursing at NR and then e-mailed me with the same information I received at eight thirty this morning.

I called the pharmacy that delivered the medications. The pharmacist said she would check with neuropsychiatrist and get back to me.

I contacted the program spokesperson who encouraged us to move Thaddeus to NeuroRestorative. I talked to him about the problems I have had and requested a transfer or Thaddeus's departure. We talked about them giving me another patient's information, the issue with dietary, the issues with medications. Also, I told him that Thaddeus's Medicaid had stopped due to SSI medical review requesting another document.

After multiple calls to psychiatrist's office, I finally had assistance from office admin. This kind person walked to records to get someone to help me. Before she returned my call, I had a call from a nurse practitioner. She confirmed the notes written by a doctor on the first visit of the 2.5 mg increase.

The neuropsychiatrist had increased the dosage from 7.5 to 10 mg on January 2 to help him. At the time, he was having a hard time with anxiety. He would exhibit angry actions, facial expressions, and say harsh words. He was gritting his teeth in anxiety and had what the doctor called a short fuse. One month later, January 30, 2014, the doctor confirmed that the dosage was correct. He told us to come back for a follow-up on April 23 (three months later).

She agreed with me that the increase was from January 2 and that she saw nothing in the notes to support 12.5 mg of Zyprexa dosage. She told me she would send a corrected script to the pharmacy and contact NR to stop the dosage.

I called the pharmacist back and told her what I had learned. She said she would have NR stop the dosage and wait for the paperwork to be sent over from U of L Psychiatric.

When I picked Thaddeus up at 4:00 p.m., I was given both dosage packs of Zyprexa and told that they would continue the dosage because they had no word from the pharmacist or the doctor.

Constant concerns in every direction kept me running from doctors to social security offices to pharmacies. I went to Social Security office in downtown Louisville, 601 W Broadway (courthouse building basement). Prior to departure, I spoke with someone by phone about Thaddeus not being able to get medications, physical therapy sessions, and the cancelled doctor's appointment due to his SSI disability case being in review. He had no more Medicaid.

At the Social Security office, I had to be screened and then sent down to the basement to the office. I checked in on a monitor at the entrance near the security desk. The number 17 was called by window 2 admin, and she told me that someone would call me by name. I waited and prayed over those who were waiting around me, thinking that none of us probably wanted to be there.

When my name was called, the person heard my case and promptly stated, "There is nothing we can do for you." I gave her my ID and then asked if she would look up his information in the system. She consented. She said that she could send a message to SSI that they take steps to urgently make a decision since his Medicaid was stopped. Then she told me that the lady I spoke with that morning, Mrs. Brown, had already sent the message. She sent me to the Medicaid office at 908 W Broadway.

I walked the three blocks in the swirling wind and went into a back entrance to a checking desk. They called my number (39) and sent me to the Medicaid floor (third floor, left of the elevator). I checked in there and was called by name to meet with Denise.

The representative heard my story about Thaddeus and began processing ObamaCare via Kynect. This would enable him to have insurance until KY SSI disability declared him disabled and reinstated his Medicaid. She told me that he would have a number by Monday. This would get him medical care.

When I went to pick up Thaddeus at NR, I asked him to give me his Well Care Insurance card given to us by KY Medicaid in November. I explained to them that this would be his insurance for the next few months until SSI disability was approved. The lady who took the card to photocopy informed me that they had a hard time getting paid for services via Well Care. I explained that this was all we could get right now. She continued to say that they had never been paid for his services at NR. I disagreed with her by saying that Thaddeus's case manager at NR, had informed me the bill was paid in full through January 31. She hissed off to talk to the case manager and returned to me without mentioning anything. I asked her if the case manager confirmed the information, and she shyly responded yes.

Last night, I finished preparing a very detailed spreadsheet workbook on all expenses and banking transactions for Thaddeus since July 1. I had to give an inventory account to the Fayette County Mental Health judge for sixty days after receiving guardianship. I listed the expenses we had personally spent for Thaddeus. He has a bank account from which I write checks for his rent at the NeuroRestorative residence. Also he received money on a US DirectExpress card set up for me by Social Security.

Today I had an appointment with our attorney in Lexington. I had previously sent over a soft copy of the Excel workbook. He had told me to bring a copy with me. At his office we reviewed the request from the court for a sixty-day inventory. Also, he had received a letter from the Department of Family Services with a statement that $154,031 was billed against the estate for Thaddeus. This was for Medicaid, and if he earned any income, it would be debited to repay this debt.

I listed that Thaddeus had $200 in clothing and personal effects plus a $69 watch I had given him. He had no personal property, including real estate or vehicles. Also we attested that he had $765 in cash on hand. No appliances, no income, no life insurance policies. We typed up the form and went to the mental health office at the court house. I was sworn to truth by the admin, who was a notary, and the document was signed and submitted.

February 23, 2014

We live in a world today where we feel entitled. According to our upbringing in the '60s to '80s, we were told that if we want something, we have to work for it. Putting all the positives in our lives and avoiding evil at all costs would guarantee a positive outcome.

Traumatic brain injury, head injury, disability, guardianship, NeuroRestorative are just a few of the words that are revealed in the next few pages. My son was hit by a car. That is enough to create pages of dramatic concern as a mother. The story I am writing is still going on. This is what you call a living document in that each day it changes.

I thought I was entitled to good things. As a young mother, my husband and I decided I would stay home and care for our children. "God first, family second, and everything else next" was my motto. Sometimes you set your plans in life, and then a major change comes along.

Yesterday, I once again left my son in the care of several qualified professionals at a program where he can learn to be independent again—whatever that looks like. Walking away from him is hard every single time.

What if he never gets well? What if he gets well and goes back to his lifestyle of sex, drugs, and alcohol? What if I have spent all this time with him and there are no changes except he needs constant medical care? It is not my health. It is not my battle. It is God who called me to this phase of Thaddeus's life. How can I move forward when I feel so defeated? How can I move forward when it is so hard to face his needs? I come home and feel defeated. I go there, and the battle rages.

Good news from University of Louisville Music Therapy. Thaddeus met with two of the therapists from U of L for the music therapy assessment. Everything went well. He responded positively when the therapist had him sign an intellectual property document.

March 7, 2014

Today I took Thaddeus to the physical therapist, Francoise. She was so comprehensive and took special care of Thaddeus. He had been cut off from his physical therapy because of the Medicaid issue. We dealt with it on my last visit—or at least I thought so. As went the trend, over the last 8.5 months about the time I think I had figured things out, they were confused again.

Yesterday, I understood that Thaddeus had to have pure Medicaid. This is an interesting term given to me by the case manager for his Acquired Brain Injury waiver given by the State of Kentucky. Pure Medicaid along with the ABI waiver allows for glasses, occupational therapy, physical therapy, and other services offered at the NeuroRestorative Facility.

Last visit (February 18–21), I was sent to the Medicaid office to reinstate his Medicaid. They told me Thaddeus had to have Well Care. Under the new ObamaCare laws, Medicaid has to be managed by an outside insurance agency. Since Thaddeus is under deferment by Social Security Disability, they had to reinstate something to give him medical coverage.

The ABI waiver case manager worked with KY Medicaid to cancel his Well Care Insurance given at the Kynect office at Medicaid so we can go forward with the full coverage that allows him to stay at NeuroRestorative. There is an old song from the '80s that has a lyric that goes, "Will it go round in circles, will it fly high like a bird up in the sky . . ."

I took Thaddeus to meet with his physical therapist. He had several problems stemming from poor control of his trunk, and his shoulders were starting to bother him. She asked me about his vision therapy.

Also, she wanted to know why he didn't get therapy at NR. They had received approval for further treatments from Well Care (eight sessions).

Thaddeus went back for behavioral therapy at 1:00 p.m. He had speech therapy from 2:00 to 4:00 p.m. I'd be back at 3:50 p.m. to pick him up. Then we would go to eat and pick up his clothes.

Thursday, March 13, 2014

I flew in from Palm Coast late last night on Delta. The last flight I could get so I could spend time with Asa and still be here for Thaddeus this morning. The winds were rough, but the pilots made excellent choices, and my travel was uneventful.

Thaddeus had an appointment with Advanced Vision for vision therapy. Today was his second appointment. The testing was completed for him back in January. He has many vision issues that are challenging him. the certified physical therapist was able to help Thaddeus with understanding the differences between shapes, letters, patterns, and light. He would go back next Tuesday.

The visit with the neuropsychiatrist was effective yet redundant. Oh well. At least Thaddeus had the right medications, and his progress continued to be good. The SSI had ordered a neuropsychological evaluation, which is done by a psychologist. I was guessing that his behavioral therapist could not perform such function. We moved his follow-up appointment to May 23.

I am weary from these things. Knowing Thaddeus needs help is tough. Knowing he is in the right place for now is good. Yet I am thinking that with no spiritual guidance, he will not be given the right focus on God. Then that is God's hand to work out this detail. I must commit to pray more and allow all things to work together for good for Thaddeus.

March 18, 2014: Thaddeus Update

We are thankful for all following our family journey through Thaddeus's brain injury.

Thaddeus made steps forward and then double steps back—this was to be expected at this point of his recovery. I just spent the weekend with him, and he slept most of the time. During my previous visit one week before, he was alert, and we had great conversations. Thaddeus was still unaware of his deficiencies. This would take time. Please pray for his strength to maintain a positive attitude and understand God's plan for his life.

He recovered from the abrupt medicine changes. In his case, less medication is better. This was one of several problems I had to deal with. Most of the issues had calmed for the moment.

His gait issues had improved. He was able to incorporate the left side while walking. One of his big challenges to physical therapy was not being able to see. Vision therapy became a must!

He was now going twice a week to vision therapy, where a therapist was training the muscles of his eyes. Since his right eye was blocked for so long, the muscles had shut down. He is getting better at opening that eye. The goal of his therapy is to be able to overcome double vision and increase depth perception.

One of the biggest joys over the last few weeks was the reintroduction of music therapy into Thaddeus's therapy lineup. The music therapist who worked with him in ICU, acute care, and Cardinal Hill is completing her master's work at University of Louisville. She goes to the NeuroRestorative center once per week to spend time with him.

These sessions had been very positive for Thaddeus and the students who came to help.

Generally, I was going back and forth between Palm Coast and Louisville twice a month. This gave Thaddeus assurance that we were still with him and I could take him away from the program for a few days—very necessary! Prayers because Asa and I would give up the house in Louisville in May. It has been such a blessing to be able to have a place to call home during this transition period for Thaddeus. I have to fight red tape in every direction on his behalf, including medical coverage, banking issues, program battles, etc.

Ultimately, Thaddeus will come to Florida. With the limited medical resources for brain injury in Florida, we still feel it is best that he stays in Kentucky a little while longer. We don't want him to feel abandoned. We wait for Social Security Disability to approve him so he can get full medical coverage.

Friday, March 28, 2014

Asa and I arrived in Louisville yesterday at noon. We took a taxi to the house to get our car. We had to take Thaddeus to his 2:00 p.m. medical appointment with a new ENT. We found Thaddeus happy to see us and not quite sure why we were there. He and Asa sat in the car while I worked with the staff to pick up medications (they have to be counted out individually) and arrange for his vacation from the program.

Tomorrow we would be traveling by van to Palm Coast, Florida, for spring break. Holton and her friend, Alton, and Thaddeus were going with us! We were so excited. We prayed for travel mercies.

Thaddeus had made some positive progress over the last few days. He had perfectly normal hearing except for some minor loss in the left ear—the doctor declared it to be hereditary. His posture seemed to be improved, and he was able to keep his right eye open more often. I asked him about that, and he said, "I can remind myself to open my eye when I realize it is closed."

Bravo to vision therapy at Advanced Eye Care! The sessions were paying off so well. Also, I received word from his physical therapist that he seemed more stable, and she was able to do more complicated standing, balancing, and exercise movement with him. With this, she recommended that he only go to therapy once per week.

We were still waiting on a decision from Social Security Disability. They had been "actively" working on his case since February 1. Yesterday, I received a phone call from the assessor, asking about his activity level. As soon as I mentioned one of his deficiencies, Thaddeus overheard and began to spiral out of verbal control.

We were picking up is favorite Strawberries and Cream Frappucino in the drive-through at Starbucks. I had to jump out of the backseat and head inside Starbucks to finish the inquisition (too cold to stand outside) we waited to hear.

Kentucky Social Security Disability had to declare the patient as unable to work. Once they decided, the SS administration decided the patient's needs for medical coverage. Since Thaddeus had an Acquired Brain Injury waiver, he had to have pure Medicaid, not ObamaCare. Then the ABI waiver covered any needed treatments not covered by Medicaid. Without these, the treatments stopped.

April 25, 2014

"Victory in Jesus, my Savior, forever, He sought me and bought me with His redeeming blood. He loved me 'ere I knew Him and all my love is due Him. He plunged me to victory beneath the cleansing flood." Thaddeus sang the words to this song on Easter Sunday with the congregation at Arbuckle Baptist Church, Lebanon, Kentucky, where our Ryan (Jessi's husband) is the pastor.

What victories we had celebrated over the last ten months! Yesterday I received a phone call from Social Security Administration to let me know that Thaddeus would receive benefits, including financial support and medical coverage. It has been a long journey to accomplish. I filled out paperwork in July 2013. We had a series of deferments, temporary coverage, review boards, extra review boards, coverage stop, and now, every benefit in full dating back to July 2. Thank you for praying!

In each step of recovery, we are faced with new challenges. I am happy to say that the challenges are becoming victories on every side! I flew to Kentucky and took Thaddeus to his physical therapy appointment. Francoise, his PT, did an assessment of his abilities during the one-hour session. I watched as she put him through challenges incorporating his lower body, torso, and upper body. He accomplished every goal she set for him, so he graduated from physical therapy!

The next steps moved him toward accomplishing normal life tasks. He would continue his speech-language pathology therapy, psychological therapy, occupational therapy, life skills therapy, vision therapy, and learn how to live independently over the next months and years. He would stay at NeuroRestorative rehabilitation for a little while longer. As he becomes more able to perform adult daily-living skills, he will move toward independence. We will then be able to bring him home.

What does Thaddeus think about all this? In his words, "I am working hard every day." "I don't like it here." "I want to be with my family." He was able to participate in a group day camp outing where he spent time outdoors with other clients at NeuroRestorative. The reports I have from the team are very positive. Thaddeus hasn't told us about this yet.

June 2, 2014

Many continue to ask us about Thaddeus. We are thankful for the continued faithfulness to pray and support us in this journey. It had been eleven months since his accident. We will start to know what normal looks like in about six more months.

He continues to make positive but slow improvements in the NeuroRestorative program in Louisville, Kentucky. He is becoming more aware of his deficiencies. This creates a new level of frustration for him. The therapists are giving him more challenging tasks to help him gain steps toward independent living and normal life. Vision therapy and music therapy continue along with the therapy program at the facility.

We are thankful for the improvements and continue to pray for his ability to cope with the new challenges he faces. Asa and I are now traveling back and forth from Kentucky together. I became so weary from all the drama and months of concern. It has been good to be together.

Yesterday we had a shocking message that Thaddeus's thirteen-year-old daughter, Holton, broke her right leg (femur near the knee). She was at a friend's house, completing a forward flip on a trampoline, and fell into the springs. She was rushed to the ER and then transported to University of Kentucky hospital. This morning, she had successful surgery. Please pray for her healing. It was unsettling for all of us.

We will start bringing Thaddeus to Florida for home visits on a regular basis beginning June 14. He had graduated from physical therapy. As he moves beyond other therapies, we will start to consider his departure from the NeuroRestorative program in a few months. God's mercies are new every morning.

July 9, 2014

Yesterday Thaddeus had two medical appointments. I wanted to take him so we could discuss progress and assure communication between the doctors.

When we saw the physiatrist, Thaddeus was very sleepy; he didn't say much to the doctor. When asked a question, he responded openly and with complete eye contact. At points, he phased out of the conversation when I was speaking with the doctor. The doctor reviewed his medicines, observed his responses, and overall aspects of grooming, posture, responsiveness, and verbal communication.

Just prior to the visit, I had played one of Thaddeus's videos from when he was at the rehabilitation hospital. He was singing, playing the guitar, and making up song lyrics on the spot while seated in his bed.

We continue to fight battles of short-term memory loss and ammonia levels that shoot high and are hard to control. The overmedication has stopped, and we are seeing Thaddeus come slowly back to us. Each aspect of the journey is long and hard. The steps forward are always followed by challenging steps. There are months of therapies and treatments ahead to know what normal will be for Thaddeus.

July 31, 2014: Thaddeus Update

Thaddeus is still continuing his daily therapies at the NeuroRestorative facility in Louisville, Kentucky. His progress is steady as he begins to become more aware of where he is and what is going on in his life. We contacted him today, and he was able to talk about the changes in his medication.

After two weeks of blood work, his liver enzymes were still elevated. His last doctor visits proved that he was overmedicated. The medications were causing Parkinsonian symptoms. A decision was made immediately to change the schedule of medicines and reduce dosages. We were pleased with the medical care he was receiving at this time. Doctors were working with the facility to get things under control.

Of course, he is anxious to get out of the program. Our plans are to move him to Palm Coast to complete his recovery once he graduates from all therapies. It takes so much energy for him to work day by day. We are starting to see some signs of normal life. Asa and I would travel back to Kentucky next week and give Thaddeus a break from the program.

August 6, 2014: Thaddeus Update

Asa and I travelled to Lexington to spend time with Thaddeus. He was able to get out of the NR home for the weekend and visit with family. He is more active and beginning to respond to questions. The therapists have been working with him on understanding how people react in conversation and also how to make conversations.

I was disappointed because he had been allowed to smoke in the facility. He had no tobacco products in his system for over thirteen months and has no dependence on nicotine. When I asked Thaddeus, he said that he was a smoker. I guess his memories of being a smoker were coming back. He had some unusually agitated behavior. I was told that his ammonia levels had increased tremendously. I wondered if there may be a correlation between the smoking and these levels. No answers from anyone.

His physiatrist has put him on treatment to lower the ammonia levels in his blood. This has been an ongoing issue since we were at the rehabilitation hospital. Somehow the testing for it didn't seem necessary. When I looked up on the Internet the reasons for elevated ammonia levels, I found lots of information related to certain medications. The elevated ammonia levels means that his body is putting a lot of protein into the bloodstream. This can cause agitation and personality changes.

Wow! That explains a lot about his behavior. Thaddeus had been angry with me. He would grit his teeth and get in my face. He perceived loving gestures to be acts of violence. He would get impatient and was always repeating the same things. He said that I was making him stay in the NR program as a punishment. He didn't want to shower, shave, or sit up with us at home.

We scheduled a trip to Florida for the Labor Day weekend, and I was hoping these levels are under control. Also, with his medication changes and his therapists focusing on his perceptions, maybe he would calm down.

In order to stop the smoking and restrict tobacco products, I learned that there is a very long process. Three explanations to get to the true reality made me very impatient with the staff at NR. They requested an emergency meeting at the facility. There we were able to hear from his therapists on his progress, and I was able to get the tobacco usage restriction on paper.

Meanwhile, I had to depend on Thaddeus to decide that smoking is not good for him. He was being treated for severe gum disease that was caused from smoking and not taking care of his teeth for so many years. Also, I explained to him that it is important for the healing of his vocal cords and his progress in speech therapy to not smoke. Thaddeus still had problems with swallowing. He had problems with reflexes in his throat. His voice is still healing—monotone with very little inflection.

At first, Thaddeus persisted in saying he needed to smoke. I prayed that God would help him to make the right decision on his own. His speech therapist spoke with him about the dangers of smoking. He took some of the words she told him and some of the words I told him and made them to be negative and verbally perseverated for days about them. He would banter at me for over an hour about me asking him to stop smoking.

Then, in a calm voice, he said, "Mom, I think I need to stop smoking. Maybe I can get some nicotine patches." I relaxed—the battle was over.

The next day in the meeting, his behavioral therapist drew up a document outlining the disadvantages of smoking and giving the program personnel permission to stop him from using tobacco products. She showed everyone, including Thaddeus. He read a little bit of the document, and then she sent around a signature page for all therapists, the case manager, Thaddeus, and me to sign, restricting him from tobacco products. He signed it!

The doctor ordered nicotine patches. He truly doesn't need them because there is no physical dependence on nicotine. Emotionally, he felt he must have them. So he had been on them for two weeks.

August 28, 2014: Picking Up Thaddeus for the Trip to Florida

I picked Thaddeus up from his home at NeuroRestorative. We had a gracious reunion. He was angry at me for leaving him there at first. Within minutes, that subsided, and he was happy to see me. He realized that I was taking him away for two weeks. He put his own bag in the car and was ready to leave. I was so happy that he seemed better. He was not angry with me, and he was not saying abusive things.

He was calmer. He seemed more alert. He was watching entire movies. I was so relieved to see this improvement. He went with me to Georgetown, Kentucky, to help Holton get her passport application. She was so happy to have her daddy with her!

We went to see Jessi and her family. He slept while we were there but still seemed to be in a happy mood. Thaddeus is getting better. He still can't remember things from his past. One day, he will remember a person, and then if I ask about them the next day, he doesn't remember. It is as though his thoughts circulate through the memory files in his brain.

We flew together to Florida, and he enjoyed the trip. He seemed excited to be home. And we looked forward to him being able to spend time with us.

September 7, 2014

Since he has been in Florida, Thaddeus seems to be having a good time. He has gone to church with us, he goes out to eat with us, and he enjoys his meals. He likes to help me cook a little. He sat on the beach for a while the other day. We went shopping for clothes, and he picked out what he wanted to buy.

He asked his dad to take him driving. Asa took him to a farm road in our Jeep and let him try to drive. He was able to do it but still has some slowed reaction times. We see progress. We are not at the end of the journey. Several months ahead will help us to know exactly where Thaddeus is going to stabilize. We pray he makes a full recovery.

The drama is less intense. The days are becoming more normal. I still travel between Palm Coast, Florida, and Louisville, Kentucky, every two weeks. We still have a home we rent from the church where Thaddeus can stay with me for the week or weekend when I am there. My life is not normal by any stretch of the imagination. I have afforded myself with some personal time to do things I enjoy.

After a conversation with my doctor, I am a little depressed and weary from the journey. I have a strategy to clear my head and refresh my heart. God has given me great strength in this journey. I enjoy my newfound business of selling Living Lockets. My fitness classes are going well. I even have some new clients looking forward to my help.

God is the one who controls the time. His plan for Thaddeus involves us. We want to be with him. We love him. We want to help him get set up again in life. He asked us in the beginning when he first started to speak, "I just want to be with you and Dad and learn the things you taught me as a child. My eyes are wide-open." We pray we can help him accomplish his goals in life.

September 11, 2014

The trip to Florida was great for Thaddeus, Asa, and me. It went by way too quick. When we reminded Thaddeus last night that it was time to head back to Kentucky, he was upset and surprised. He didn't remember that he was supposed to go back today. It's tough.

It was pretty dramatic for a while, and he just decided to go to bed and deal with things tomorrow. Sadly I knelt by his bed to pray. Taking him back is very hard for me too. We know it is the right thing to do—it is just so hard. We, like Thaddeus, want things to be normal again. Unfortunately, we don't even know what normal is supposed to be.

We packed and readied for the trip. I have to carry his medicines in my carry-on bag, so we have to go through extra screening at the airport. They test the vapors of any liquids. We were able to take advantage of boarding first, so Thaddeus had time to walk down the jet bridge. I am always thankful he can walk. There are so many who are dependent on wheelchairs to get to and from the plane.

Flying over the ocean, we looked at the coastline and thought about the next trip we would make to Florida next month. Each month, we want to bring him home to see how he does. In this trip, he was able to go the beach one afternoon, out to eat many times with us, and even to church once. The best part of having him here is the smiles on his face when we do things together. He watched several movies on TV; we made regular trips for cheesecake and movies. It brings a smile even now to think about it.

Thaddeus has doctors, therapists, and activities in Louisville. In Florida, we have to find a way to create these for him. It will take a lot of prayer and work to assure his medical coverage in Florida to set up new doctors and therapists. I wish it would happen soon.

As I finish this book, please know that we are still waiting to see what normal is going to be for Thaddeus. He wants to be independent. I want him to be independent. The time is in God's hands. With all the right therapies, medicines, and positive motivation we can get for Thaddeus, God will bring him to what he wants Thaddeus to be.

Your loved one will come back to you too. It may take a lot longer than Thaddeus's journey, but then it could be a lot less. Please take time to do everything you can to facilitate the recovery. Don't be discouraged when it seems your efforts are failing or unusually unappreciated. Keep understanding that the waves of recovery are sometimes overwhelming and sometimes peaceful. Like our doctor told us, this is a "marathon and not a 5K."